Speak Up and Stay Alive

SPEAK UP
AND STAY ALIVE

The Patient Advocate
Hospital Survival Guide

Health & Happiness

Pat Rullo

PATRICIA J. RULLO

MILLENNIUM STAR PUBLISHING
CHAGRIN FALLS, OHIO

Copyright © 2012 by Patricia J. Rullo
Millennium Star Publishing
46 Chagrin Plaza #103
Chagrin Falls, Ohio

For information regarding special discounts for bulk purchases, wholesale, or private labeled books, contact msp@millenniumstarpublishing.com

To book the author to speak to your group or organization, visit the website: www.speakupandstayalive.com or contact: speak@speakupandstayalive.com

Printed in the United States of America
ISBN: 978-0-9799807-6-3

Contents

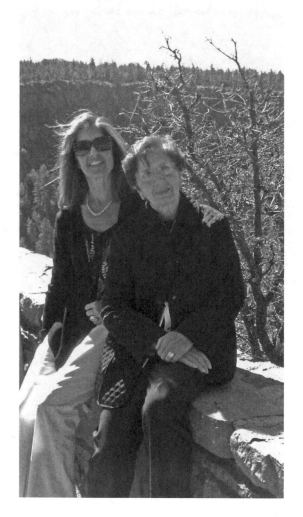

Grand Canyon, Arizona

Dedication

To my mom.
Your experience was a gift and a lesson
to everyone around you.
Thank you for surviving.

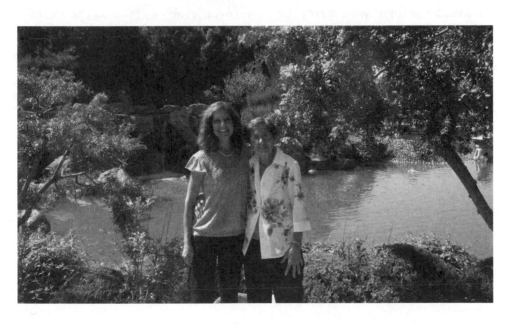

Japanese Friendship Garden, Phoenix, Arizona
One Year Later

Disclaimer

THIS book is not about bashing doctors, nurses, hospitals, or the health care industry. Although hospital safety statistics are alarming, hospitals do more to help than they do to harm. The majority of doctors and nurses are amazingly dedicated people who surrender their lives to do exhausting work to help others in need. Most patients leave the hospital with their problems solved, ready to take on the world as functioning individuals.

The health care system is also fragmented, and many patients are compromised. I hope this book changes your frame of reference and gives you permission to insist on having someone intelligent advocate and navigate for you. Do not be afraid to know your rights, to stand up for them, and to take action. Please read this book with the understanding that the author, publisher, and all parties involved are not rendering any medical, health, legal, or other professional advice or services; they do not intend to replace professional medical care and expressly disclaim all responsibility for any liability, loss, risk, or injury resulting from the use and application of any of the contents of this book, public speeches, presentations, or safety logs associated with this book, or any content taken from the book's website - www.speakupandstayalive.com.

Preface

"**I** challenge you to be your own advocate." A wise nurse attempting to tell us something without actually saying it offered this advice to my mom about three months into her hospital ordeal. The enormity of her words hit me as a blast of freezing-cold air. She knew the faults of the system. She knew that if we did not try to save ourselves, we might not make it. Until that instant, I did not realize that by participating in every routine and every seemingly insignificant nuance of my mom's care, I was acting as her advocate. And I had every right to advocate for her because she was not able to speak up for herself.

Until that nurse issued her challenge, I had been acting on instinct. From that moment on, I used her words as a green light. I accepted the challenge, took the lead, and continued to demand explanations, justifications, and proof. I became an active participant in the fight for my mom's life.

Thanks to my Latin studies, I am fascinated by the origins of words. The word *patient* comes from the Latin word *patiens* and translates to "someone who suffers." As an adjective, the word means "to bear or endure without complaint." The word has chilling synonyms: invalid, uncomplaining, long-suffering, forbearing, resigned, passive, and calm. Should we really behave as patient patients? Do the submissive-sounding synonyms set the stage for their unconscious fulfillment?

The word *advocate* comes from the Latin root *vox*, which means "voice," making a patient advocate the voice of someone who suffers. Perhaps we should empower ourselves with a bolder, more proactive title. I do not want to merely be a voice; I want to be an activist—a direct participant who takes action or effects change, someone who is involved, effective, and physically energetic and who exerts influence. As much as I prefer the motion associated with the word, activist, I use the term advocate throughout the book, because it is commonly recognized and accepted. The bottom line is—a hospital stay is no time to be a weak voice in the background. Use this book not only as a guide but also as a personal challenge to become your own advocate or an advocate for a friend or loved one in need. If you choose to accept the challenge, this book will give you the tools you need to become an intelligent health care consumer.

Get ready to become a speak up and stay alive patient or advocate.

Acknowledgments

As always, I am thankful for Bob—my best friend in life. He quietly took care of everything while I stayed at the hospital. Each day as I ran out the door before dawn, he handed me lunch, snacks, water, and extra cash. He kept my car filled with gas, did the laundry, paid the bills, made special late-night dinners, and let me cry as much as I needed. I could not have been there for my mom had he not been there for me.

My niece, Kate, lived with us and was a bright spot during a gloomy time. At the end of each day, she greeted me with a clean house, her smiling face, and a warm hug. When Mom came home to our house, Kate stayed up all night for weeks to be on call so I could sleep. It was one crazy summer and having her with us made all the difference in the world to me.

Christine, my daughter, was my long-distance support. Her phone calls let me know I was not alone. Despite her hectic work schedule, she came to town on several occasions to accompany me on my hospital vigils. Both Mom and I valued those soft and silent times as three generations prayed for a miracle.

Finally, I thank the intelligent, kind, and supportive doctors, nurses, and other hospital staff who helped us survive those dark days with their keen surgical abilities, their wise decisions, and their willingness to talk, comfort, and care for our family. I will always respect and honor them.

Introduction

MOM'S cardiologist gently grasped my arm in the hospital hallway. I did not know him, and his visit was unannounced. In a hushed voice, he asked me to join him in a small room just outside the cardiac intensive care unit where Mom was fighting for her life. As the door closed behind us, another door opened, leading me into a world of fear, anger, disbelief, and—ultimately—strength.

Dr. Kay was Mom's primary cardiologist. He had learned through the hospital network system that she had suffered a serious myocardial infarction after shoulder surgery. Two days after her heart attack, he took it upon himself to find me to share information that he asked me to keep confidential. As he handed me a yellow envelope, he said, "This stinks, and you need to do something about it."

Ten days earlier, Mom, who was seventy-eight years old, fell while working at a bridal shop. While retrieving a veil for a customer, she tripped over a two-inch-high threshold between the stock room and the showroom. She fell forward, absorbing the full impact with her shoulder. The city had cited the faulty threshold as a building violation long before the shop opened for business. It was one of many violations the shop owner felt free to ignore. The city also chose to overlook the violations and permitted the shop to open to the public with unchecked and unresolved safety hazards. Because the accident happened at work, the incident was reported to the Bureau of Workers' Compensation. To add insult to the injury, the shop owner had not paid the premiums in over a year. With no coverage in place, the owner was liable for all medical bills. A little string pulling, some political mumbo-jumbo and a check for eight hundred dollars put the shop owner in the clear. It makes me wonder why any employer would bother paying Workers' Compensation premiums. However, that is another story for another time.

The fall crushed Mom's right shoulder. Repairing it called for surgery. The surgeon recommended a reverse total shoulder replacement, a unique procedure that switches the ball and socket. It is a highly technical surgery in which a metal ball is attached to the shoulder bone, and a plastic socket is attached to the upper arm bone.

Mom was scheduled for surgery on the following Monday. After we arrived at the hospital, the staff prepared her for surgery. We waited for four hours until they sent us home because the surgeon "didn't feel well." Interestingly enough, as we headed out of the hospital, I saw the surgeon getting off the elevator, drinking a cup of coffee, and laughing with another doctor. They strolled out, talking and joking around. I am not a doctor, but he didn't look sick to me. After three days of stressful attempts to reach the surgeon, and cryptic conversations with his not-so-helpful secretary, they rescheduled the surgery for Thursday.

Mom was feeling ill the day before the surgery. We chalked it up to nerves, yet looking back, she may have been showing signs of a heart attack. On the morning of the procedure, during the presurgery assessment, Mom's blood pressure was 80/55. She complained of not feeling well. The assistant anesthesiologist (who, incidentally, had his license suspended a few weeks later for stealing anesthesia drug waste to support his own drug habit), looked at the head anesthesiologist with concern in his eyes and asked her, "What about the blood pressure reading?" She ignored him.

The surgeon walked in and asked to view the preoperation test results from the X-rays and electrocardiogram (ECG) Mom had taken a few days earlier. They were nowhere to be found. His secretary had failed to forward them, despite several phone calls from me and the lab to request that she do so. The surgeon laughed and blamed it on the lab, saying, "That's the Greenfield lab for you."

Despite Mom's warning signs, the shoulder surgery took place. I sat in the waiting room from 5:30 AM until 10:15 AM, when the surgeon came out and said that Mom was in recovery and I could see her in forty-five minutes. Eleven o'clock came and went. I watched the surgeon and his assistant leave the hospital and enter the parking garage. At noon, I questioned the woman at the reception desk, and she told me Mom was in "pain management."

Finally, at 1:15 PM I was allowed to enter the recovery room. Mom's skin was pale gray. She complained repeatedly, "I don't feel good. I don't feel good." When asked where she felt pain, she pointed to her chest. With that, one of the nurses gave her an injection of Versed, a sedative that stopped Mom's words before she could complete the sentence. The last thing I heard her say was, "I don't feel..." and they sent me out of the room.

At 3:20 PM, the receptionist called me back into the recovery room. Seconds later, the nurses ushered me out. At 4:30 PM, a nurse came out to the waiting room with an anxious look on her face. "Your mother is having a heart attack, and we have to get her to the operating room as soon as possible," she said. The staff scrambled once again to find the preop ECG results to use as a comparison, however thanks to the indifferent surgeon and his secretary, the prior test results were not there.

If not for Dr. Kay, who risked his job and his reputation to share his findings with me, I would not have known what actually happened the morning of Mom's surgery. Based on the nonchalant attitude of the surgeon and anesthesiologist, I was suspicious of their desire to complete the surgery, yet nothing prepared me for what was inside the yellow envelope.

As we sat at the small conference table, Dr. Kay showed me a copy of the ECG taken two days earlier, at 10:53 AM the morning of the surgery. It showed not only the squiggly lines on the rhythm strip, which as a layperson I did not understand, but written at the top of the page were the words, *heart attack in progress*. He then showed me the results from the follow-up ECGs taken around 1:00 PM, 3:00 PM, and again at 4:20 PM. All of them showed clear signs of heart trouble.

At 10:53 AM, a heart attack was in progress, which means she had likely been having heart trouble before that, perhaps even during surgery. At 11:00 AM, the surgeon had sauntered out of the building, either unaware of the heart attack or not caring about it because his part of the job was over. In addition, an entire post-surgery unit's staff and anesthesiologists had failed to recognize and follow up on what should have been obvious to any medical professional.

In the days and weeks that followed, it became apparent that the hospital was well aware of the potential for a wrongful death lawsuit if

Mom were to die. They bent over backward to offer special treatments and proposed a surgery not ordinarily performed on a person of Mom's age. This salvage surgery involved a seldom-used procedure using a right ventricular assist device, performed by an outstanding surgeon.

They gave Mom the only closed-door private room in the intensive care unit. Everyone was doing everything possible to keep her alive. I was in an interesting position in that I knew all the details of the undiagnosed heart attack, and yet no one knew that I knew. This allowed me to observe behavior, watch body language, and have pointed conversations with subsequent surgeons, doctors, and hospital staff. I took this time to gather information to complete the facts surrounding the grievous mistake.

So began four months of Mom's repeated brushes with death—all because of human error, ignorance, and carelessness on the part of the hospital and its staff. I witnessed many adverse events during Mom's experience. Several resulted in formal hospital-documented incident reports. Certain staff members were prohibited from entering Mom's room. For example, I watched a surgeon attempt to insert drainage tubes to remove fluid that was accumulating in Mom's chest. In the process, he punctured one of her lungs, causing blood and fluid to spray around the room. Another doctor ushered me out, but I remained in the hallway, watching as at least a dozen nurses ran in and out of the room with blood transfusions and other lifesaving devices. To make matters worse during these frantic moments, the power went out, sirens blared, and a lockdown mandated through the public-address system. The convergence of these events set the tone for the incomprehensible trials we faced on an almost daily basis.

A week later, a friendly but overly talkative nurse "accidentally" administered epinephrine (also known as adrenaline) instead of the intended drug, the antibiotic Vancomycin. The mistake was noticed, not by the nurse, but by my daughter just before Mom went into cardiac arrest. Meanwhile, every few days the shoulder surgery anesthesiologist, who was mainly responsible for the missed heart attack, and her assistant, would surreptitiously peer into Mom's room while exchanging furtive and knowing glances with each other. They were not a part of Mom's care team and had no reason to be hanging around her room.

They had no idea I knew about the life threatening error or that I kept a watchful eye on their suspicious rounds.

The shoulder surgeon made it a point to be unavailable. Eighteen hours after Mom's shoulder surgery, she was back in the operating room for her second heart surgery. I ran into him in the hospital hallway. Nervously he offered, "Oh, I just saw your Mom a few minutes ago. She looks good." I answered, "Really? Where did you see her? She's been in surgery for the last five hours." I was shocked that he so freely lied to me. Throughout the rest of Mom's stay, his absence and elusiveness continued. Every Friday, Mom's doctors, surgeons and nurses held a family meeting to keep me informed of her progress. Each week I requested his attendance. Each week he phoned in with an excuse. One evening I saw him enter the ICU. I crossed his path and asked him directly what went on during the morning of Mom's shoulder surgery. He danced back and forth, slipped his shoe on and off and said, "Had I known what I do today, I would have done things differently. The anesthesiologist didn't tell me your Mom was having a heart attack." His body language and ambiguous answers left me knowing there was more to the story. I never saw him again. He didn't return—not even to remove her stitches. Four months later, a nurse at the rehabilitation center noticed nylon threads hanging from Mom's shoulder. She removed them herself while shaking her head in disbelief.

For weeks, mom needed a ventilator to help her breathe. She was *intubated* with an endotracheal tube inserted through her mouth. The tube was tied with thin straps around her face and taped into place on her cheeks. Bound and gagged, she looked like a prisoner. The pressure from the straps caused serious skin breakdown to her lips. She was unable to speak or move and was groggy from drugs. In an effort to communicate, I recited each letter of the alphabet until she stopped me with a slight eyebrow movement that I often missed. Sometimes this spelling exchange took hours and made it difficult for me to understand her concerns. One morning, through this obscure method of dialogue, Mom indicated pain at her urine catheter site. All day I begged the nurse to change it. She always had an excuse. At the end of the day, as I headed toward to the exit door, I saw the nurse waiting in the hallway with the new catheter package. I turned around to see her enter Mom's room, so

I headed back. I watched, and it became clear why she had not changed the catheter while I was there. She obviously did not know how to do it. She unfolded the directions that accompanied the tubing kit and placed them on the bed. Then she turned the tube in many directions, trying to match the pictures on the paper. When I noticed that she was not wearing gloves, I popped in and asked her to send a nurse who was qualified to change a urine catheter.

Early the next morning, I entered Mom's room to find her feet bound with bloody gauze. I unraveled the gauze and saw all ten of her toenails, mangled and torn as if someone had used a machete to cut them. I flew out of the room to the nurse's station to demand an explanation. For some reason, a local podiatrist had made his rounds in the middle of the night to perform his ghoulish "pedicures." "Oh yeah," one of the nurses responded, "we get complaints about him all the time." I promised them that if Mom got an infection, I would take serious measures to address this heartless and macabre action.

Two weeks later, my mind was shattered once again as I watched a senior physician teach a roomful of interns how to clean a bedsore. As the students gathered at Mom's bedside, the doctor wandered across the room to the windowsill where I kept my Clorox wipes. (Each morning I wiped every surface in the room in an attempt to keep the germs at bay.) Somehow the doctor had spotted the wipes, and before anyone could react, he pulled several out of the container and proceeded to wipe the bedsore with Clorox bleach. The hospital filed another incident report, and the doctor was banned from Mom's room. These are only a few of the bizarre and unimaginable events that took place right in front of me. I can only wonder how many other mistakes occurred when I was not there. However, despite the constant calamities—many extremely competent doctors, nurses, and hospital staff eventually saved the day.

Throughout this experience, I had the opportunity to feel fear and enter the unknown, and emerge as a wiser medical consumer with a message to share. When life presents difficult assignments, I always ask myself, "What am I supposed to do with this information?" This book is my answer. If my mom's experience helps one other person, then there is a positive reason for her journey.

I now travel from state to state—speaking to groups, organizations, and companies—to create awareness and help build educated and empowered hospital safety support groups within those groups. In addition to the book and personal presentations, a comprehensive set of safety logs serve as a supplement. The logs help you track and monitor everything from doctor and nurse visits, medications, questions and concerns, vital signs, and contact information. It also includes a hand washing reminder sign, a list of common hospital terminology, and much more. These safety logs are real-time tools to help you stay organized and safe during a hospital stay.

The best way to survive a hospital stay is to stay out of the hospital. However, if you find yourself faced with a hospital visit, I encourage you to take this book and the safety logs with you. Use them as a guide to remind you of ways to protect yourself. Give copies to your friends, family members, and coworkers. The information in this book applies to everyone. Learn how to be your own advocate. Try to have an advocate with you at all times during a hospital stay. Better yet, offer to be an advocate for someone else. There is no richer reward than helping another human being survive.

CHAPTER 1

Advocates and Awareness

A hospital stay is a stressful time. Emotions run high. Anxiety and fearfulness become normal. Good judgment takes a back seat. Decision making is delegated to those who don't know you. Doctors take charge, and you let them. A place you believe is safe is peppered with pitfalls. Disease and discomfort seize the day. You are not at your best, and you are in no position to watch for hospital health dangers. You need a bodyguard—someone to step in to look out for your best interests to bridge the gap between you, your doctors, and the hospital staff. You need a communication steward. You need a patient advocate.

The National Patient Safety Foundation answers the question, what is a patient advocate: "An advocate is a supporter, believer, sponsor, promoter, campaigner, backer or spokesperson. It is important to consider all of these aspects when choosing an advocate for yourself or someone in your family. An effective advocate is someone you trust who is willing to act on your behalf, as well as someone who can work well with other members of your healthcare team such as your doctors and nurses" (2003).

You can make use of several resources to implement a culture of advocacy during a hospital stay. Usually an advocate is a family member—a spouse, parent, child, or grandchild. The need to have someone present around the clock is crucial, yet sometimes it is not feasible. Most family members have other obligations including work, school, or parenting and cannot take months, weeks, or even days off to live in your hospital room. One solution is to have appropriate candidates work in shifts or rotations. Employ a sign-up sheet with dates and times and have family members commit to a schedule. Assign one person as the lead advocate through whom all communication flows. Log everything in the safety logs that supplement this book to track and monitor all important information.

If family is not available, ask a friend, neighbor, coworker, or church member to help. Using a rotating schedule, find someone to act as coordinator and rally the troops to sign up for times. Again, assign one person as the lead advocate to avoid chances of miscommunication.

Another option is to hire a sitter. This person may or may not have a medical background. It is helpful to have someone who understands hospital lingo and protocol, yet it is not crucial. You want someone who cares about your outcome just as you do. Have a friend or family member inform the community that you are looking to hire sitters to stay with you during your hospital visit, or ask the hospital staff if they know of any independent folks who do this. Many times the nurses know of these people through former patients who employed hired sitters to act as their personal advocates.

Another option to use in conjunction with a family, friend, or hired sitter is a private, professional patient advocate or a health care navigator. Karen Morrisey, a health care consultant and patient advocate who owns Golden Navigator in Scottsdale, Arizona, explains how this option works:

> There is a lot of discussion these days in regards to the "sandwich generation" and it can go both ways, with children assisting parents or sometimes grandparents assisting with grandchildren or their own children.

> I am hired either by family members or directly by the client. Often family members are out of town, and the patient realizes he or she needs help. Sometimes the patient won't listen to family members but is receptive to an outside perspective based on facts not driven by emotions. Also, there always seems to be one family member, usually female but not always, who is the responsible person. If this person works full time, he or she may not be able to "do it all" or may not be knowledgeable in health care issues.

One client found me when a friend referred her to the National Association of Healthcare Advocacy Consultants website. She called, and as she described her situation, I felt confident I could help her. I suggested we meet in person, as I do with all of my clients. We met for two hours, and she talked nonstop. I explained how I could help her, and we departed, leaving her to contact me if she wanted to get together again. She called thirty minutes later and hired me.

She has been in and out of the hospital a half dozen times in six months. This included emergency room visits as well as surgery. During her hospitalization, additional heart problems surfaced, and she was referred to yet another specialist. At this point, her primary care physician "lost patience with her and her questions." She was confused and did not know what to do next. Various doctors ordered tests and changed her medication without really listening to her. She was also new to Medicare and confused about her plan and needed guidance regarding alternative programs. She needed someone to listen to her and point her in the proper direction so she could have the under-standing about her changing health. We worked together to find a good, compassionate primary care physician who was in her insurance plan's network. Now she feels better and more in control of her conditions and understands she has as voice. She is "empowering" her team of medical professionals to attain the best health possible. She knows I am here when she needs me and can contact me at any time. (Morrisey, pers. comm.)

Insurance does not cover the cost of private health care navigators or advocates, so you are responsible for any fees. These folks offer many valuable services and can save you thousands of dollars, if not your life. A private advocate has knowledge of the health care system or has a medical background. Advocates who provide medical assistance can help you find an appropriate doctor or surgeon; locate nursing homes or specialty treatment centers; review your diagnoses and treatment options; help acquire and review medical records and test reports; assist with discharge; accompany you to doctor appointments; or stay with you bedside during critical times.

A private advocate not only knows the health care ropes and offers unbiased suggestions; he or she also cares to understand you as an individual. Much of health care is non-relational. Doctors and hospital staff have little time to develop a sense of who you are or what you need on a human level. Carol Cusick, a patient advocate and owner of C. Cleary Cusick, Inc., in Tarrytown, New York, exemplifies the much-needed relationship side of health care.

A woman named Ida was scheduled for exploratory surgery and she asked Carol to accompany her for moral support and to act as her advocate. When diagnosed with ovarian cancer, Carol helped her understand the doctor's prognosis and care recommendations, coordinated her chemotherapy and radiation treatments as well as her home health care. To maintain Ida's well-being and peace of mind, Carol managed the insurance claims and prescriptive schedule. She worked to ensure that Ida's home was comfortable and safe to accommodate her newfound medical state.

After a period of treatments, Ida went into remission and began to live life again. She enjoyed her hobbies, especially dancing and going out with friends. During this time, Carol kept up with Ida's check-ups and medical maintenance as well as the insurance claims and appeals. Sadly, the cancer came back and was more challenging this time around. Carol continued to act as an intermediary between the doctors, interpreting their recommendations and pressing for further clarification when needed. With her help, Ida enjoyed the remainder of her life without the worries of tending to insurance and medical bills—tedious details that often overshadow patients and deprive them of important quality time to enjoy life. She was comforted to know that Carol was not only her advocate, but also her friend.

Your patient advocate isn't your only health care advocacy resource. Health insurance and hospital billing issues can be overwhelming. Understanding your insurance plan can be difficult. An advocate trained in this area can help you choose an insurance plan; analyze medical bills

and look for errors and overcharges; file or dispute a claim; or negotiate denials. It's important to ask questions before the service to avoid
surprises when the bills arrive. Will you pay extra if specialists are not
covered under your plan? Patricia Ruminski, the owner of Medical Cost
Control Inc. in Calimesa, California tells of her recent hospital experience. She illustrates the need for a patient advocate on several levels:

> My husband was dying of cancer. I was his primary advocate.
> With my knowledge of medical billing and experience as a
> medical administrator, I tried to stay on top of things. Our insur-
> ance paid 100 percent of all charges after our deductible, as long
> as the providers were members of our PPO. My job was to make
> sure every doctor who treated my husband was a member of our
> PPO. I learned the difference between the doctor who "accepts"
> the PPO fee from the doctor who is "a member" of the PPO.
> The costs could be huge if a non-member saw my husband on
> an ongoing basis.

> My husband's cancer eventually spread throughout his body,
> bones and brain. While receiving brain radiation, a psychiatrist
> came to visit with him. I asked if he was a member of our PPO.
> He said he would bill our PPO. Clearly, this did not answer my
> question. After some prodding, he told me he was not a member.
> Because I wondered about the value of psychiatric evaluations at
> a time like this, I asked one of our specialists to stop the psychi-
> atrist appointments. The next day the psychiatrist showed up
> again. I told him nicely that since my husband could not commu-
> nicate, there was no need for his services. Later, the specialist I
> initially asked to halt the psychiatrist visits, stopped by to thank
> me. He said, "It's difficult for one doctor to fire another one and
> I am relieved that you did it." Had I not been there to monitor
> this situation, no one would have questioned the rationale for
> the psychiatric visits, our specialist would not have intervened
> for fear of professional impropriety, and we would have received
> expensive out of network fees. (Ruminski. pers. comm.)

Insurance and medical billing aren't the only challenges. Navigating through legal matters is not something you can do on your own. Legal issues are complex. Common sense does not always prevail. A lawyer versed in health care can help draft advance directives or he or she can assist with disability issues, worker's compensation, or medical malpractice.

The hospital patient advocates or patient representatives can help you. They work for the hospital as part of the risk management team. They do not work for you; they work because of you and only as it pertains to their job description. They can help with certain hospital-related questions, can cut through red tape, and know where to refer you for additional resources. This option is not an option for your day-to-day and hour-by-hour safety.

The smartest way to ensure a safe hospital visit is to combine all of these advocacy resources. Have a lead advocate who knows you best and can spend the biggest chunk of time with you. Use sign-up sheets for family and friends to commit time to relieve your main advocate. Hire additional help as needed. Use a professional patient advocate to guide you through the confusing health care maze, and use the resources the hospital offers.

To locate a patient advocate, visit the following websites. They offer free search options by location. Once you narrow your options down to your area, you can then contact them directly:

- National Association of Health Advocacy Consultants (NAHAC): (www.nahac.com)
- AdvoConnection (www.advoconnection.com)

There is no formal certification training or credentials for patient advocates. It is up to you to interview and screen your candidates to make sure you and your family are comfortable with them. Ask key questions:

- What is your background, training, and credentials?
- What other situations have you handled in the past? What was the outcome?

THE PATIENT ADVOCATE
SPEAK UP AND STAY ALIVE
HOSPITAL SURVIVAL GUIDE

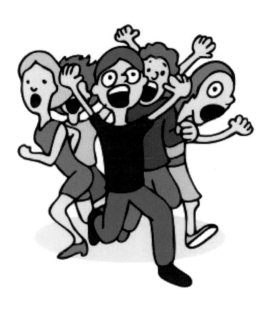

PATRICIA J. RULLO

www.speakupandstayalive.com

Speak Up and Stay Alive

Schedule a presentation
that will save your audience
from little known healthcare
and hospital hazards.

With Pat Rullo -
your survival guide and
nationally recognized author,
speaker, and radio hostess .

Fun, fast paced, and
jam packed with serious
information.

And as always -
Pat delivers with a light touch
of humor and wit.
Your crowd will love it!

speakupandstayalive.com

pat@speakupandstayalive.com

440-725-5462

- Do you have the background and time to handle my case?
- How are you paid?
- May I contact recent references?
- Do you live nearby?

How to be an effective patient advocate

If you hire a sitter or a professional advocate, look for appropriate advocate traits. You may not have this luxury when using a family advocate. Even among non-family candidates, your choices may be limited, making it unrealistic to find someone who knows how to get along with people or who has the personality or stamina for the job. If you do have a choice or if you are an advocate reading this book, here are suggestions that make for an effective patient advocate.

It is possible to be an advocate without alienating hospital staff. You do not want to get in the way of any important tests, treatments, or procedures that might save your patient's life. Being an advocate is all about being informed, present, persistent, and caring. It is not about being loud, arrogant, adversarial, or obnoxious. A little humility and willingness to be a team player are key. Although it is good to be suspicious of all things, keep that position to yourself as you quietly look into everything and anything that may need your attention. No one needs to know what is really going on in your mind until you take action.

If possible, have your patient introduce you to the doctors and nurses in charge. Let them know you will act as an advocate and to allow your questions and concerns as if coming from the patient. Dress well. Dress for success. Dirty sweatpants and sneakers do not exude power. When you look important, people take you seriously.

Some staff members may view you as a nuisance. Some may appreciate your efforts and others may feel threatened. Don't let this attitude scare you from your duties. You are not there to validate yourself. You are there to save a life.

Do not talk negatively about doctors or nurses in any public places. And don't talk about one nurse to another.

Understand your patient's wishes in the event of a life support event. Read and review all signed advance directives with your patient, including living wills, power of attorney or health care power of attorney paperwork, organ donation forms, and do-not-resuscitate orders.

To minimize the chance of conflicting orders from specialists, have one doctor coordinate your patient's treatment. Ask the name and title of every caregiver. Ask how they fit into the caregiving team. If you feel this is too forward, tell them you want to know so that when you need help in the future, you won't waste their time calling for an inappropriate reason. Write down their names, and use them when speaking to each person in the future. Everyone likes to hear his or her name. Show you care by remembering and using their names.

Establish meaningful relationships with the doctors and nurses. Try not to pull strings for minor problems. Ask for their help by using the words "help" and "can you help me understand?" and conclude any service—a bedpan request, a bath, or a pillow fluffing—with the words, "thank you for helping me" or "thank you for helping us." People want to be helpful, and they appreciate a sincere thank-you. It makes them feel good. However, if you ask for help on several occasions with no resolution, ask to speak to the hospital's patient advocate or social service worker.

Practice a little personality style awareness. Quickly assess the personality style of each doctor or nurse. If your doctor speaks hurriedly and to the point, don't attempt to chat about sports scores. Get to the point quickly and succinctly. If a nurse is chatty and friendly, take time to ask questions and get to know him or her. Be aware of the differing personality styles of your health care team, and deal with them in the ways they prefer to communicate.

When the doctor pays a visit, listen first and then ask your most pressing questions. Have a prepared list. Don't waste his or her time with useless questions or conversations. Doctors always have one foot out the door, so prioritize your questions and get to the point quickly.

Gain valuable allies. If staff members share personal information with you about their children, weekend plans, hobbies, and such, use this as a way to make friends. On Monday, ask about their weekend and inquire about the child's softball game. Building relationships is an important skill to hone during a hospital stay. Find common ground, and share something personal about yourself. If a doctor, nurse, or aide considers you a friend, you will get better treatment. Who would ignore the needs of a friend?

When you go to the cafeteria for a snack, ask your nurses and aides if they want something. Occasionally bring a box of donuts, a bag of apples, or other goodies as a way to say thank you. A little schmoozing never hurts.

Know the time of day the doctor or team makes rounds. This tiny amount of time holds an entire day's worth of information. Find out the plan for the day, any medication changes, test results, or changes in diagnosis or treatment plans. Your patient may be asleep or groggy. This is your time to shine.

Frequently the food on the meal tray is not compliant with the patient's diet. Or if the patient is asleep when the tray is presented, the staff may leave the food out of reach. Your patient may not eat if the food gets cold or if no one is available to retrieve the tray or help with feeding. Malnutrition is one of the top hospital risks. Make it a point to have someone available for all meals unless your patient is fed intravenously. Patricia Ruminski tells a mealtime story with serious implications. "My husband was also diabetic and needed insulin before he ate. The food-staff delivered his meals bedside. Due to the brain tumors and brain radiation, my husband was forgetful. Yet he was expected to know if he had been given his insulin. Many times, I had to remind the nurses to furnish the insulin prior to the meal. Because his case was complicated and required many specialists, I saw how difficult it was for more than one doctor to treat him. The computer systems did not make it easy for the doctors or nurses to get a clear picture of the case because they did not have access to each other's data. This is likely due to privacy regu-lations, but made it difficult for them to provide seamless care. As his advocate, I was there to ensure continuity and fill in the blanks when necessary."

As an advocate, you can help prevent these kinds of things from happening—simply by being present.

In addition to mealtime mistakes, shift change is a highly dangerous time—a time when the patient or the advocate is not included in the process. Miscommunication and errors are common when those who are leaving are anxious to get home. The new shift is inundated with new information about several patients. Mistakes happen during these "handoffs." As an advocate, use this time to inform and remind the new shift of any important changes, observations, or circumstances surrounding your patient. Do not expect a seamless transfer. Stick around to make sure everyone is on the same page. If you cannot be there, leave notes on the bed tray and call a few hours after the shift change to make sure the new team is well informed. Watch for deviations in care—skipped medications, missed or inappropriate meal trays, or forgotten baths.

Help the nurses with simple routine care. When housekeeping arrives, ask for extra towels, washcloths, bed linens, blankets, and a pillow. Or ask where the fresh linens are stored and get permission to retrieve them. Keep a stash in the room so you don't have to call for a nurse. Reserve a drawer for extra napkins, straws, plastic silverware, bandages, transfer pads, and other routinely used items.

Stay with your patient during all trips out of the room, including gurney or wheelchair visits to radiology, testing, or procedures.

Changes in vital signs are often the first sign of an upcoming problem. Ask for the results each time vital signs are taken. Record them in your safety log for future reference. What might be a normal vital sign reading for one person may not be normal for someone else. However, medically safe ranges exist. If any vital sign rises or falls more than 20 percent, ask for another reading with a different piece of equipment. Monitor any reading that remains high or low. If a vital sign changes more than 40 percent of the normal reading, get immediate help. Here are the safe ranges for the most frequently monitored vital signs:

- blood pressure: 90/60 to 120/80
- breathing: 12–18 breaths per minute
- temperature: 97.8–99.1° Fahrenheit
- pulse: 60–100 beats per minute—usually measured with a finger clamp called a pulse oximeter or a "pulse ox"
- oxygen saturation: 90–100 (Oxygen saturation readings assess a patient's need for oxygen, measured with the finger clamp oximeter. A reading under 85 is cause for concern.)

Question new medications before allowing your patient to take them. Check IV and blood bags for correct patient name, and ask the nurses to explain how to understand pump settings and decipher monitor settings.

Make sure the staff wears gloves during any procedure that involves needles, blood, tubes, incisions, or open wounds. Watch for good hand hygiene. If a nurse or staff person shows signs of a cold or cough, you have every right to request another nurse. Ask if anyone on the floor has MRSA, an antibiotic resistant staph infection, or C diff (a bacteria with airborne spores). If so, ask what protocol is in place to prevent your patient from getting these nasty bacteria. To prevent the spread of these dangerous germs, hospitals may provide single-patient use, disposable blood pressure cuffs.

Ask your nurse to combine all blood tests into one blood draw. Activities including bathing, dressing, therapy, blood pressure, temperature, and weight taking can also take place at the same time. You and your patient deserve a few hours of uninterrupted rest. You can also request that testing take place during daytime hours.

If visitors get too numerous, too frequent, or too noisy, it is up to you to create and enforce the boundaries. You may not be popular for the decisions you make, but popularity is not in an advocate's job description.

What may seem unimportant today may become a pivotal piece of information in the future. That's why it is a good idea to keep copies of test results organized in one folder. Use the safety logs to keep track of everything that happens.

Germs and bacteria can find you too. Be a clean freak. Wash your hands and use hand sanitizer religiously. When you get home, leave your shoes outside, change clothes, and wash your hospital clothes. Bacteria can live on fabric, and you don't want to bring any nasty germs home with you.

Keep a list of emergency numbers with you at all times. This includes phone numbers for your patient's family, friends, and doctors. Bring and use your own pen and keep paper in your pocket for quick note-taking.

Just about the time you try to sneak over to the cafeteria, something may come up that mandates your presence. Hospitals may allow you to order a food tray for a small price. Pack healthy mini meals, snacks, and water. Hydration is important, especially in a hospital setting where the air may be dry. Each floor has a small kitchen; ask if you can get water and ice for yourself or your patient, or bring your own. For further comfort, keep a sweater or blanket and a pillow in the room because sometimes the heating and cooling systems are erratic.

It's important to take care of yourself. Find a time when your patient is sleeping or when rounds, medications, and baths are over, and go outside into the fresh air. Or you can wait until visitors arrive and use it as an opportunity to take a walk. Do deep breathing, yoga, or tai chi. Remember, it is important to recharge and refuel.

To help pass the time while your patient recuperates, bring your laptop, books, or relaxation music with you. Research, research, research. Use the Internet to look up medication names, diagnosis, and treatments. Become educated and use your new knowledge as needed.

Being a full-time advocate takes its toll by disrupting your work and family life, and it may add financial pressures and drain your mental, physical, and emotional reserves. You cannot do everything by yourself. Ask for help and accept help. You will not be useful to your patient if you burn out. Share your feelings with others. Talk with other advocates or join a caregiver support group. Whatever you are feeling is valid. Be kind to yourself.

Finally, an advocate's job is to ensure continuity between people, departments, and facilities. Every hospital department, floor, or wing is its own microsystem, or culture, where the staff works together for a similar purpose, using particular equipment and procedures to treat patients with similar problems. Because microsystems are unique little entities and are fairly independent of the larger system, it can be difficult for one system to seamlessly link to another. This rift can cause fragmentation of care. In a hospital setting, patients move from one system to another, for example from cardiac surgery to intensive care to rehabilitation. The handoffs or transitions between these microsystems or departments can be dangerous. Quality of care can change as it crosses into a new microsystem, and vital information can be miscommunicated or perhaps not communicated at all. It is important to recognize this lack of cohesion as you travel between these systems.

When you are sick and in a strange place, you may not have the awareness to think about microsystems, handoffs, and communication mishaps. To this day, my mom has no idea what happened to her during most of her four months in the hospital. When I tell stories, she shakes her head and says, "I must have been out of it. I don't remember that at all." While she was "out of it," I was "in it," watching everyone and everything, questioning, reading, researching, and coordinating. That is the job of an advocate.

CHAPTER 2

Prepare to Prevail

Legally

As my dad used to say, "Make sure your house is in order." In other words, take care of the legal issues you may be putting off. Take some time to execute, copy, and distribute the following documents to appropriate family members. In addition, the hospital will ask for copies, yet these documents are not required to receive care in a hospital. It might cost a few dollars to prepare them, however the cost of not having them can be devastating to you and your family.

Medical Documents

An *advance directive* is a document that gives directions in advance about your future medical or surgical treatments. A living will and a durable health care power of attorney are two important advance directives. According to a recent National Center for Health Statistics Data Brief, only 37 percent of older adults have an advance directive, and a mere 5 to 15 percent of all adults, regardless of age, have an advance directive (2011). These shocking numbers suggest that people are uninformed or simply choose to stick their heads in the sand. Either way, it's not smart.

A *living will* is a written, dated statement that directs health care providers to either allow or refrain from utilizing medical or surgical treatments should you be in a terminal condition as confirmed in writing by two physicians. Treatment measures—dialysis for kidney failure, a breathing machine if you can't breathe on your own, tube feeding if you can no longer eat, or CPR if your heart and breathing stop are examples of such medical treatments. A living will has nothing to do with your personal property, bank accounts, or real estate. It does not give anyone the right to make decisions for you. It simply states your health care wishes.

A *durable power of attorney for health care decisions* is a written document in which you designate another person as your attorney-in-fact to make health care decisions if you are unable to do so yourself. These health care wishes are stated in your living will. Most people use their state's standard forms, however the verbiage may not say what you really mean to convey. Before an emergency strikes, take time to review several different forms to ensure that the documents you sign represent your true meaning and intent, and that they are valid in your state.

A DNR or a *do not resuscitate order*, is another kind of advance directive. A DNR is a request to forego cardiopulmonary resuscitation (CPR) if your heart stops beating or if you stop breathing. Resuscitative methods include chest compressions, electric heart shock, artificial breathing tubes, and special drugs. Doctors and hospitals in all states accept DNR orders and you can revoke a DNR at any time.

Nonmedical Documents

A *durable power of attorney* or *financial power of attorney*, permits the person you designate to handle your finances should you become incapacitated and can no longer make decisions for yourself. When you create and sign a durable power of attorney, you give another person legal authority to act on your behalf when it comes to finances—not health matters. Without this document, your family will have to deal with court authorities to handle your financial affairs. This could be a time-consuming event, filled with red tape and aggravation.

Specify that you want your financial power of attorney to be *durable*. If you don't, in most states it will automatically end if you later become incapacitated. The word *durable* means that the power of attorney will still be good even if you become legally "incapable." The durable power of attorney will contain words saying, "this instrument will survive my incapacity." The powers you give to your attorney-in-fact will remain effective even though you may no longer be able to give instructions.

Or you can specify that the power of attorney does not go into effect unless a doctor certifies that you have become incapacitated. This is called a "springing" durable power of attorney. It allows you to keep control over your financial matters unless and until you become incapacitated; then it springs into effect. Again, you must specify that you want your power of attorney to be durable. If you don't, then in the case of a springing power of attorney, your document will never take effect at all. Take the time to create these documents ahead of time. Each state may have a different law, so be sure to have someone well informed assist with the preparation.

A *last will and testament* is a document that details the distribution of your property, money, and belongings after your death. In the document, you also name a representative (called an *executor*) to distribute your property in accordance with your written wishes. A will is a complex document, and it varies from state to state, so have an experienced attorney help you with the preparation, execution, and recording process.

You do not want to die *intestate*. When you die without a valid will in force, you die intestate. Without a will, the distribution of your remaining assets becomes the responsibility of a probate court. When this happens, a court-appointed executor—someone whom you do not know and who never knew you or the relationships you had with your family members—compiles all of your assets, pays off any lingering liabilities, and then distributes the remaining assets to those considered your beneficiaries. The problem with this, of course, is that the wrong folks may end up with the contents of your estate instead of those you would have wished.

A *life insurance policy* is the most important investment you can make. It allows for tax-free and hassle-free wealth distribution among your beneficiaries, making it the easiest and most economical way to facilitate financial and emotional security to your loved ones. It allows remaining spouses to grieve without financial pressures, families to remain in their homes, children to go to school, businesses to transfer quickly, and it solves just about any other financial situation you can think of. For pennies on the dollar, you can save and protect your family members. If you don't have a life insurance policy and are relatively healthy, contact a reliable life insurance company to discuss and implement the options that work best for your circumstances. Can you tell how I feel about the beauty of life insurance?

How to Select Your Health Care and Financial Power of Attorney

Most people name their spouse, their partner, a relative, or a close friend as their health care and financial power of attorney. That is fine if you are certain you can trust this person with your life. Discuss ahead of time your feelings and wishes about your financial situation, potential health care needs, and end-of-life issues. Feel certain that this person will respect and honor your choices, even if he or she doesn't agree with them.

A Few More Things to Consider

A power of attorney has the potential for power, so give it to the right person. Do not feel forced to select someone just because he or she is a spouse, child, or relative. If this person is in any way immature, emotionally questionable, disinterested, scared, financially broke, unemployed, or shaky in any other way—select someone else. To smooth things over, tell this person that you are not going to select them because they could be too emotionally connected to the situation and you don't want to put them in that situation. This is not the time to play favorites or placate someone.

When driving a car, only one person can step on the gas. If two people sit in the driver's seat, expect a crash! Likewise, only name one person as your power of attorney. It is a good idea, however, to name alternate agents in case your main person becomes unable or unwilling.

In a perfect world, your daily hospital advocate should be your health care and financial power of attorney. Your advocate will know every detail of your condition and have the best background when making health and financial decisions for you. What you don't want is your health care power person pleading for medical help and your financial power person saying no or dragging his or her feet. But life is not always perfect, so choose your people well by putting the best person in the right job. If you feel that you must name two different people, make sure they know each other and can get along. If your health care power of attorney lives halfway across the country, make sure that person agrees and is willing and able to spend weeks and months with you at the hospital. It could be difficult for a long-distance person to make wise choices based on a few phone calls. If you do not have anyone who satisfies the critical criteria of assuming the power over your health care, do not name anyone. Your living will requires your health care providers to follow your written wishes. So at the very least, prepare a living will and discuss it with your doctors so they are aware of your desires. Ask them if they are comfortable with your directions and if they will in fact honor them. If they express any reason at all that they may not be willing to honor your choices, ask them to direct you to a doctor who will. This is not the time to worry about making waves. Your life is at stake.

The person you select must be self-assured and firm. On several occasions, I faced last-minute judgment calls when the nurses called the entire family to Mom's bedside to say good-bye. Certain family members tried to push me to make quick end-of-life decisions. Fortunately, I stayed on my path and was not inclined to waiver from what I knew Mom would choose. And thank goodness I was strong, because Mom survived and is living a nice life. So when choosing an advocate, pick a person who is not worried about winning a popularity contest.

How to Get the Job Done:

Although you can go to the Internet and download forms, you may want to work with an attorney. He or she can provide you with the correct state forms, notarize and record any document that may need recording, and hold a copy of your documents in their files for safekeeping. Alternatively, here are other ways to write your advance directives:

- Write your wishes by yourself.
- Ask your doctor or hospital to provide some of the forms.
- Contact your health department or state department on aging to get certain forms.
- Download the forms from the Internet.
- Use a computer software package for legal documents.

Whichever way you decide to prepare your documents, make sure they comply with your state laws. Keep the original copies of your advance directives where you can find them. Give a copy to the person you've named as your health care proxy, to your hospital advocate, and to your doctor, hospital, ambulatory surgical center, nursing home, or other health care providers. Also carry a card in your wallet that states you have advance directives. The point is, just do it.

Mentally

Why feel helpless and frustrated when you can be intelligent and empowered? Your goal is to make educated choices. Study up on everything pertaining to your situation. Read this book a few times. Underline parts you want to remember. Share the book with your family and chosen patient advocate so that everyone understands how to avoid hospital pitfalls.

Choose an advocate. It could be a family member, a friend, or a hired sitter, companion or health care navigator. Make sure everyone is on the same page. Your mind will be eased to know that you won't be alone and that someone who cares for you will look out for your best interests.

Before a hospital stay, listen to relaxation music or subliminal health recordings. Feed your mind positive, healing thoughts.

Physically

If a hospital stay is in your future, you and your immune system need to be strong enough to ward off infections, effects of stress, disease, and exhaustion. Now is the time to get in shape or stop smoking. Learn tai chi or yoga. The breathing techniques alone can increase your stamina.

Nutritionally

It is especially important to ramp up your nutritional status before a hospital stay. If you know you will be admitted to the hospital, imme-diately start to eat healthy foods, including lots of fruits and vegetables. Include good quality nutritional supplements, protein, and probiotics. Skip the alcohol, sodas, candy, chips, and other junk. Build up your nutritional reserves with foods that will help you, not kill you. Buy a juicer and juice organic carrots and other high-powered vegetables in an effort to mainline the nutrients. Juicing is a quick and easy way to saturate your system with powerful vitamins and minerals needed for healing.

Spiritually

Spirituality is a private matter. You do not have to be a religious person to be spiritual. Before a scheduled hospital stay, read books or listen to CD's that reinforce your belief system. Bring them with you to the hospital so you have something familiar and safe from home to fall back on.

Study new philosophies. They say when the student is ready, the master appears. I've noticed that during particularly trying times in my life, I seemingly stumble upon something new that suddenly sheds an illuminating light on my problem. This new information causes me to look at my troubling situation in a new and positive way.

Emotionally

It's normal to be nervous and anxious prior to a hospital stay. That's why preparation is important. You may feel less emotionally charged when everything else discussed in this chapter is in order.

Finally – Pack a Bag

Even if you don't have a hospital stay looming in your future, pack a hospital bag ahead of time. Keep it stashed in the closet in case you have an emergency and have to get to the hospital in a hurry. Or perhaps you might get a sudden call to help a loved one, a friend, or a neighbor who needs someone by his or her side. Either way, you won't be thinking straight. How helpful would it be to have everything you need just waiting for you? A family member can always bring extra necessities as the days go by, however sometimes that may not be possible.

Essentials include the following items: infection protection items including an unopened and large canister of disinfectant wipes, a bottle of hand sanitizer gel, and a pack of disposable gloves. Other items include a wireless computer or other Internet device so you can research unfamiliar medical words and diagnoses; toothpaste; a toothbrush; a comb or brush; a razor; a nail file; a Chapstick; your favorite face or body soap; deodorant; hand or body lotion; an extra pair of drugstore glasses; copies of your driver's license, medical card, doctor's contact information, list of current medications (names and dosages), and emergency contact information; an extra pair of underwear; lipstick and other makeup; a bottle of water; a snack; gum; mints, and your *Speak Up and Stay Alive* safety logs.

If you implement all or most of these preparation strategies, you can concentrate your hospital efforts on getting well and getting out. Remember, when disaster strikes, the time to prepare has passed.

To help ease the burden of preparing your hospital bag, our website offers a ready-made Infection Protection Survival Bag. It is filled with vital necessities for your safety and well-being: www.speakupandstay-alive.com

CHAPTER 3

Remember Your Rights

As a patient or an advocate, be aware that you have rights. Although to have those rights respected, you must know what they are. Often, the hospital gives you a copy of these rights in conjunction with privacy policies and other administrative papers—that most people never read. Upon admission to the hospital, you have more important things to think about, right?

If you know your rights, you will feel comfortable in asking and making sure those rights are respected. Just because you have the rights does not mean that during your visit, a doctor or nurse will not attempt to strong-arm you into believing that you have to do what he or she tells you to do.

The bottom line is that you retain all rights over what happens to you. Your right to accept or refuse treatment is protected by constitutional and common law and by the federal Patient Self-Determination Act (PSDA). You can refuse treatment, you can refuse to have a specific person treat you, and you can insist that your surgeon perform the actual surgery instead of a resident.

My mom and I took advantage of those rights. We had a particularly obnoxious intern who randomly popped into Mom's ICU cubicle and shouted scary diagnosis thoughts. I called a family meeting and had the intern banned from Mom's room. Another afternoon an obvious beginner tried to figure out how to insert Mom's chest tube drains. He fumbled and huffed as he repeatedly attempted to jam the pigtail catheter into her skin. To my surprise, Mom chased him out of the room. Protecting your rights is up to you—and your advocate.

The American Hospital Association (AHA) approved the first hospital bill of rights in February 1973. Years later, they changed the format to a brochure called *The Patient Care Partnership*, which similarly informs patients about what they should expect during their hospital stays— high quality hospital care, a clean and safe environment, involvement in your care, protection of your privacy, help when leaving the hospital, and help with your billing claims. The addition of the word *partnership* attempts to lessen the former dogmatic approach and says to everyone involved that patient care is in fact a partnership.

Here are a few patients' rights from *The Patient Care Partnership— Understanding Expectations, Rights and Responsibilities*:

What to Expect During Your Hospital Stay
High quality hospital care. Our first priority is to provide you the care you need, when you need it, with skill, compassion and respect. Tell your caregivers if you have concerns about your care or if you have pain. You have the right to know the iden- tity of doctors, nurses and others involved in your care, and you have the right to know when they are students, residents or other trainees.

A clean and safe environment. Our hospital works hard to keep you safe. We use special policies and procedures to avoid mistakes in your care and keep you free from abuse or neglect. If anything unexpected and significant happens during your hospital stay, you will be told what happened, and any resulting changes in your care will be discussed with you.

Involvement in your care. You and your doctor often make decisions about your care before you go to the hospital. Other times, especially in emergencies, those decisions are made during your hospital stay. When decision-making takes place, it should include discussing your medical condition and informa- tion about medically appropriate treatment choices. To make informed decisions with your doctor, you need to understand: the benefits and risks of each treatment, whether your treatment is experimental or part of a research study, what you can reasonably expect from your treatment and any long term effects it might have on your quality of life, what you and your family will need to do after you leave the hospital and the financial consequences of using uncovered services or out-of-network providers. Please tell your caregivers if you need more information about treatment choices.

Discussing your treatment plan. When you enter the hospital, you sign a general consent to treatment. In some cases, such as surgery or experimental treatment, you may be asked to confirm in writing that you understand what is planned and agree to it. This process protects your right to consent to or refuse a treatment. Your doctor will explain the medical consequences of refusing recommended treatment. It also protects your right to decide if you want to participate in a research study. (2003)

The Joint Commission, an independent nonprofit group that accredits most of the hospitals in the United States, now requires all hospitals to have a bill of rights. Most hospitals tailor this document to best suit their facility and cater the text to the dynamic of their community. A copy of these rights is given to each patient or parent upon admission and it must also be posted at entrances and other prominent places throughout the hospital. Be sure to ask for your hospital's version of patient rights and responsibilities. Read it, and keep a copy in your room for reference.

Informed Consent—Your Right to Know, Consent, and Refuse

In addition to receiving a copy of the bill of rights, you will be asked to sign an informed consent form, which entitles you to know and understand everything pertaining to your treatment. You have the right to accept or refuse. Once you sign it, the hospital has the right to treat you. Before you sign, you should fully understand the risks, the rewards, the probable results if you decline treatment, the alternatives, the basic procedure, the likelihood of success, any potential complications and side effects, the recovery process, and if the procedure is covered by your health plan.

If possible, have your advocate with you when you sign the informed consent form so that someone witnesses that you signed before any anesthesia. Do not feel rushed. Read the document carefully before you sign. Do not be afraid to ask questions if you don't understand any details included in the form or if it doesn't fully explain everything you want to know. Do not sign any open or blank release forms. Your advocate may be thinking more clearly, so be sure he or she reads the form with you. In fact, you or your advocate may want to read it aloud. Patient safety is a team effort. By working with your doctors, nurses, and other health care staff, you can make your hospital stay as safe as possible.

CHAPTER 4

Pick Your Providers

CHOOSING a primary care doctor is equal to choosing a health care mate. He or she should know you and your health issues, and show concern for them too. This person acts as the main coordinator of your care. He or she performs your regular wellness checkups, tends to routine or sudden illnesses, refers you to specialists, and should be the one medical person you feel is in your corner and has your best interests in mind. That is why you should choose this person with care.

Besides a primary care doctor, your situation may dictate the choosing of additional and different primary care providers. These doctors may include internists who act as primary care/general practitioners and have further training in specialties—digestive medicine; heart specialists; OB-GYNs (obstetrics/gynecology); pediatricians, or geriatricians who specialize in health care for older adults.

Regardless what kind of primary care doctor you choose, take a few steps to make an informed decision. First, ask for referrals from friends and family. Usually if those you trust have good things to say about their doctor, it is worth pursuing. You may feel comfortable with a doctor who shares a similar status as you—gender, race, age, ethnicity, religion, or viewpoint. If this matters, narrow your selection by looking for these qualities first. Is the location convenient for you and your family? You won't enjoy an hour drive every time you or your family members are sick.

The next step is to research the doctor's education, certification, and performance history. To verify that the doctor is board certified, visit The American Medical Association website (www.ama-assn.org) and The American Board of Medical Specialties website (www.abms.org). Go to your state's physician licensing website to check for any license revocation history (www.patientsrighttoknow.org). Another resource to help find a doctor or a surgeon is the American College of Surgeons website (www.facs.org). Counties may offer information on their websites about malpractice grievances. You can usually find this under clerk of courts/ common pleas at your county website. This does not mean the doctor was guilty of any malpractice; it shows that he or she was included in a malpractice suit.

The final step is to make an appointment to interview your potential choices to discuss your health concerns to see if you feel comfortable with the answers to your questions. Don't wait until you are sick to begin this process. It may take weeks or even months to get an appointment as a new patient. Once your relationship is established, most doctors will give you an appointment quickly if your medical condition warrants.

Here are a few basic questions to help you identify a suitable choice:

- Does the doctor have the training and background to meet your health care needs?
- Does the doctor have privileges at the hospital of your choice, and is he or she a part of your health plan's network?
- Does the doctor or accept Medicare and Medicaid?
- What are the doctor's hours of service, and who covers for your doctor when he or she is not available?
- How does the doctor handle payment and cancellations?
- Does the doctor have any history of malpractice?

Once you've covered the basic housekeeping questions, then it's time to get to the heart of your selection process. Here are a few more questions you may want to ask:

- Does the doctor offer a holistic and preventive approach based on a cooperative relationship, or does the doctor know best, leaving you with little control?
- How does the doctor feel about alternative, complementary, and natural choices? Is he or she quick to prescribe pills, antibiotics, and invasive tests?

- Does the doctor explain things in a way you thoroughly understand, treat you with respect, and take the time to listen to you?
- Will the doctor share written copies of your test results with you?
- Does the doctor's personality mesh with your personality? Do you enjoy this person's "bedside manner?"

When interviewing a potential primary care physician, look for the non-tangible answers to your questions as well as the actual ones. A doctor may look good on paper, but if he or she is not respectful, you may want to look elsewhere.

Be especially observant of the office atmosphere. Is the office staff happy, cheerful, and respectful of you and others? Is the waiting room dirty, messy, or cluttered? Are the exam rooms spotless, or do you see dust on the blinds, hair on the floor, and overflowing garbage containers? The doctor may say all of the right things, however if the space is not clean and the staff is grouchy, go somewhere else.

The bottom line is how this person makes you feel. If stature, education, awards, and reputation are your main criteria, let the facts guide your decision. If personality and social relations are more important, let your instincts help in your selection. Choosing a doctor is as personal as choosing a spouse. What works for one person may not make sense for you.

Urgent or Emergency Care Centers

These kinds of facilities come in handy if you have a non-emergency medical problem during the weekend, holiday, or if you are traveling. These centers usually have long hours and are open every day. They are not a replacement for your primary care doctor, yet they are a convenient option. Many urgent care facilities are part of a larger hospital system, so your records can flow through to your primary care doctor.

To make sure your local urgent care center is adequate, stop in when you are feeling well. Make sure the center accepts your health plan. See if they are accredited by the Joint Commission (www.jcaho.org) or by the Accreditation Organization for Ambulatory Healthcare (www. aaahc.org). The certificates should be posted in the office; if they are not, ask someone at the front desk or check out the websites. Ask who owns the facility and about the training and certification of the doctors and staff. Make sure it is clean, and visit the public restroom to check for tidiness.

Choose Your Hospital

People may spend more time creating criteria and profiles on dating websites than they would ever consider when selecting a hospital. Most folks just follow their doctor's suggestion, not fully realizing that the doctor may have a financial interest in the recommendation. Just because a hospital is world renowned for cancer does not mean they are as worthy when it comes to heart-related issues. In addition, your insurance plan may dictate your hospital selection. Many matters influence your hospital choice. It is important to determine what makes sense for you and your situation.

A local community hospital can have ten beds compared to over one thousand beds in a metropolitan area hospital. The more beds a hospital has, the more services they offer. Several distinct hospital service models exist, and in the past twenty years or so, hospitals have consolidated into multihospital systems. Hospitals are classified according to the kinds of services they provide or their financial statuses (e.g., publicly owned hospitals, nonprofit hospitals, and for-profit hospitals) The majority of hospitals are nonprofit. Some for-profit hospitals are owned by large corporations. If the corporation is a public company, the hospital must pay back a portion of their profits to investors. Other hospitals are funded by the community taxes. Military hospitals, academic hospitals, and many others also exist.

General Hospitals

The most familiar type of hospital is the general hospital—no, not the television soap opera. The general hospital attends to many diseases and injuries, and usually has an emergency department. Your small local community hospital may be considered a general hospital and so can larger major health care facilities that offer departments in surgery, intensive care, labs, and so on.

Specialized Hospitals

Specialized hospitals include those that treat specific patients, including children or seniors, or they treat a particular illness. Many physicians who refer patients to specialty hospitals have an ownership in the facility. In the spirit of full disclosure, ask your referring physician if he or she has any financial ties to the proposed facility.

Ambulatory Surgery Centers and Clinics

Ambulatory surgery centers perform surgical procedures on patients who do not need an overnight stay in the hospital, and many times they specialize in a particular area of medicine such as gastroenterology or orthopedics. Surgery centers may be entirely physician owned. Others share joint ownership between physicians and private or publicly traded companies, and in some cases, hospitals and hospital networks own others.

Emergency Rooms

Hospitals specialize in different areas of medicine and this can make a difference in how you are treated in an emergency. If you have a specific medical issue, check out those hospitals and emergency rooms that cater to your needs. Some emergency rooms specialize in pediatric or senior care. Do your research before a crisis strikes. Ask if the doctors on staff are board certified in emergency medicine. What hospitals do they use if you transfer for further care? Are they open 24 hours every day of the week?

Teaching Hospitals

Teaching hospitals affiliate with universities, medical schools, or nursing schools for medical research purposes and to train medical students, interns, and residents to care for patients. Teaching hospitals also provide care to millions of uninsured patients. The advantages of teaching hospitals are many: the latest treatments, research developments, and high-tech equipment are available at teaching hospitals, which in turn attracts high quality physicians, specialized medical surgeries, and procedures. You gain the expertise from many accomplished physicians, and new up-and-comers who understand today's technology.

However, this can be a double-edged sword. The focus on teaching can result in unnecessary patient testing; eager students can contribute to wrong diagnosis; and the sheer number of staff that surrounds one patient can cause miscommunication setbacks.

Regardless of which kind of hospital you choose, check with your state's health department. Each state has a website with hospital data, quality of care scores, certifications, and types of procedures. The Joint Commission's website (www.jcaho.org); allows you to search by hospital, location, or type of service and get reports on hospital practices based on The Joint Commission's inspections of each facility it accredits. From there, visit the Department of Health and Human Services website, *Hospital Compare* (www.hospitalcompare.hhs.gov). This website allows you to search for hospitals by city, state, or other criteria; look up statistics; and compare more than five thousand hospitals against one another and to state and federal averages.

As you narrow your choices, don't forget to check with your insurance provider to see what hospitals are covered in your area. You may have to go out of network and pay more. Make sure your doctor has the ability to care for you at the hospital you choose. We were blindsided by this when Mom was in the hospital rehabilitation wing. Doctors seemingly appeared out of nowhere in the middle of the night and made medication changes. As hard as I tried to be there when they arrived, their phantom visits eluded me. After days of trying to reach them by phone, I called Mom's primary doctor to ask if he could monitor her care. He answered me as if I should have known better and said that he did not have privileges on that floor. Find out these kinds of things before selecting your hospital.

Contact the hospital directly through their risk management department to ask about their history of hospital-acquired infections, medication errors, and the other risks cited in this book. Ask about the nurse-to-patient ratio, and inquire about the RN- and LPN-patient ratios. You want registered nurses to be abundant. Tell them you plan to be an informed patient and need to gather as much information as possible. If you ask for their help with a nice attitude, you will most likely get what you are after.

If you want to dig deeper, here is a list of additional questions to ask your potential hospital:

- Does the hospital have experience and success with my illness?
- Describe my coordination of care. Is it team based, or will one doctor or nurse be assigned to my care?
- How do staffing levels change during the weekends, night shifts, holidays, or summer? Will someone of quality be accountable during those times?
- Tell me about your infection control protocol. How can I be sure not to get a hospital-acquired infection?
- What controls do you have in place to avoid medication errors, bedsores, etc?
- Can I have a private room?
- Do you welcome my advocate's presence? Does the hospital and staff welcome patient and family member involvement?
- Will my advocate and I have access to daily charts and lab results?
- Can a family member or advocate stay in my room at all times, day and night? If so, do you furnish cots or chair beds?
- What are your visiting policies and times?
- May we use cell phones, laptops, or cameras?
- What kind of security can I expect?
- Do you offer spiritual services?
- Does the hospital have a library I can use for reference purposes?
- To whom do I speak if I have a problem with the quality of my care?

Ask friends who may have stayed at the hospital you are considering about their experiences. Visit the hospital yourself. Is it within a convenient driving distance for you and your family? Wander around the halls, visit the cafeteria, and ask the hospital staff to let you see the patient rooms. Quietly check for safety, comfort, and cleanliness and observe the attitude of the nursing staff. Are they friendly and polite? Are they people you want to answer your call button? Talk to the families of patients in the waiting rooms. Most will be happy to share their thoughts with you.

If you are unsure and afraid to ask these hard yet essential questions, or if you don't have the time or energy to do the research, you can hire a professional health care navigator. Many qualified people do this for a living. They can guide you through the process because they are familiar with which questions to ask and know how to recognize the desired answers. You can find qualified names listed at the back of this book under the Helping Hands section. Finally, after your research is complete, use your gut instinct. Only you and your loved ones know what is right for you.

CHAPTER 5

Hospital Hierarchy

TO succeed in any situation, it is important to know the hierarchy. You won't be successful at a restaurant if you place your food order with the hostess. Similarly, you won't get approval for a home loan from the bank's drive-through teller. Every business has a pecking order, especially a hospital. To get help with the least amount of time and effort, it pays to be aware of the chain of command. Use this knowledge to your advantage by dealing with the correct person as soon as a problem, question, or situation arises.

Medical

Medical director—a physician employed by a hospital to serve in a medical and administrative capacity as head of the medical staff

Head of department—the physician in charge of a department of a hospital

Attending physician—the most senior doctor directly responsible for patient care

Hospitalist—a doctor employed by the hospital to care for patients in the hospital who usually does not have a private practice

Fellow—a physician who completed a residency and is training in a specialty

Chief resident—the most senior resident responsible for all other residents

Senior resident (third-year resident or above)—a physician trainee who helps coordinate the care of patients and supervises less experienced residents

Junior resident (second-year resident)—a physician trainee who helps manage patients and supervises and teaches first-year residents and medical students

Intern (first-year resident)—a physician trainee who has finished medical school and is beginning patient care duties

Medical student—a student in medical school who works with and observes the medical team

Administrator on call—a hospital executive who responds to emergencies after hours

Nursing

Chief nursing executive—a registered nurse in a management position who supervises the care of all the patients

Director of nursing—a nurse whose function is the administrative and clinical leadership of the nursing service

Nurse manager or nurse supervisor—the most senior nursing staff member, primarily administrative

Nurse practitioners, clinical nurse specialists, advanced practice nurses—a registered nurse with advanced academic and clinical experience and the ability to diagnose and manage most common and chronic illnesses; that provides care previously offered only by physicians; and that in most states has the ability to prescribe medications

Charge nurse—the nurse usually assigned for a shift and responsible for the immediate functioning of the unit; responsible for scheduling and making sure nursing care is delivered safely and that all patients in the unit receive adequate care; usually the frontline management

Registered Nurse (RN)—a bedside nurse who is responsible for direct patient care; is permitted to administer medications under the supervision of doctors; keeps records of symptoms and progress, and supervises licensed practical nurses (LPNs), nursing aides, and orderlies

Licensed vocation or practical nurse (LVN or LPN)—a nurse who has completed a practical nursing program (generally one-year-long training) and is licensed by a state to provide routine

patient care under the direction of a registered nurse or a
physician

Unlicensed assistants—nursing assistants, also called nurses' aides,
assistants, patient care assistants, or technicians

Other Care Providers

Rapid response team—a team of critical care specialists called to
evaluate a patient in an emergency

Hospital pharmacist—a pharmacist responsible for receiving,
storing, and distributing pharmaceutical supplies

Therapists—therapists who specialize in areas of speech, respiratory, occupational, physical therapy, and others

Technicians—technicians trained in specialties including radiology
(X-ray), ECG, phlebotomy (the drawing of blood), and others

Social workers—coordinators of communication, community
resources, counseling, paperwork, and discharge needs

Patient Care Advocates—hospital employees who help patients
solve problems pertaining to quality of care, safety, communication, policies, and procedures

Dietitians/nutritionists—staff trained in the use of diet to promote
health

Transporters—orderlies that move patients from place to place

Environmental Services/Housekeeping—hospital staff who provide
a clean environment for the patients and public

Because so many staff members exist, it is easy to see how mistakes
happen. That is why the patient or the advocate must know who's who.
When doctors and nurses come in and out, it is hard to keep track. To
help with this, ask your nurse about clothing identifiers. In many hospitals, the length or color of medical uniforms identify the status of the
staff. Usually the most highly trained doctors wear the longest white
coats. Because coat length increases with seniority, you can use this as a
guide. If someone in a short white coat enters your room, this may indicate a student or resident. At a glance, you know not to ask for serious
medical advice. Some hospitals do not permit white coats at all, prefer-
ring business attire because of a well-known syndrome called "white

coat hypertension"—when patients show elevated blood pressure only in hospital or doctor related settings. The hospitals that abolish white coats also believe the attire contributes to a subconscious power influence between doctor and patient. Additionally, the white coats can be a health hazard harboring and transmitting infectious diseases as doctors go from room to room or go days without laundering. In some hospitals, the nurses dress in colors specific to rank. Light blue might be for aides and navy blue for nurses. You may not remember everyone's name, but at least you may have a visual distinction. You don't need to call the RN to help with your TV remote, and you don't want to ask the nurse assistant to change IV tubing.

Warning: if you cannot identify the staff through visual or clothing cues—do not assume the nurse caring for you is a registered nurse (RN). On many occasions during Mom's stay at the rehabilitation center, there was no RN on the floor. LPNs and assistants with little experience with the complexity of Mom's medical situation often mismanaged our care. I don't know if it was a financial problem or a staffing shortage, but most days I had to stand outside of Mom's room, wave my hands, and look scary to get someone to respond to a call bell. Once help arrived, the person was harried, irritated, misinformed, and brief. Always insist the proper person do the proper job.

Rounds

The swarms of folks who circle your bed and crowd the tiny hallways each morning are the attending physician and the residents. Making the "rounds" each day is part of the attending's duties. The residents get hands-on experience with patients while following the attending on rounds. This is the last part of a resident's training to become a qualified doctor. The attending encourages resident participation in the treatment of patients and provides them with a basic daily plan of patient care. Attending physicians have final responsibility, legally and otherwise, for patient care, even though some decisions are made by others.

All of these folks can be a blessing, as many trained minds commingle thoughts, opinions, and remedies. Conversely, I saw aggressive residents try to make a name by offering unsolicited advice that proved incorrect.

A "food chain" exists inside the hospital walls. When you understand the hierarchy and call the right person for the right job, you will receive better care.

CHAPTER 6

Health Care Hazards

YOUR unawareness of hospital hazards may be riskier than the hazards themselves. To solve a problem, you need know that it exists and understand how and why it happens in the first place. That is why each risk is divided into short sections:

- what they are
- how and why they happen
- what to look for
- how protect yourself

Doctors and nurses do not go into the medical profession to intentionally damage or kill their patients. They are regular people who chose medicine as their job. Similar to your hairdresser, car mechanic, and plumber—your health care provider is simply doing his or her job. Hospital personnel have normal everyday problems and the same joys, hopes, and fears, as the rest of the world. They juggle home and work schedules, wonder what to make for dinner, and hope their children make it home safely from school. They are not any more special, deserving, or intelligent than anyone else. So why put them on a pedestal? Why do so many people fear they might look stupid by asking questions? Doctors and nurses are just people. End of story.

Every hospital has a large cast of characters. Many hospitals are teaching hospitals with an abundance of doctors in assorted stages of training, all contributing to patient care. They make bedside appearances, either individually or in groups. They rotate in shifts, making your daytime doctors and nurses different from your nighttime crew.

They often change teams. The unfortunate result is the possibility that no one is in charge. With these combinations of communication crossing paths, it's easy to see how mistakes can be made.

When you add ego into the mix, the mess gets worse. Medical specialists often vie with each other for decision-making power. If the hospital has their own hospitalists, they may have the ability to override a specialist's or primary care physician's suggestions. We experienced this disastrous setup. Mom's rehabilitation center had a roving group of hospitalists, each assigned to attend to patients one week per month. Each week Mom had a different doctor who believed he or she had a better answer than the previous doctor did. So weekly, medications were subtracted and new ones added, and old therapies were discontinued and new ones started. There was no continuity of care and no common thread, except for me. I figured out the wacky system and asked for one doctor. This decision came a little late. By this time, Mom was suffering from the hallucinogenic effects of multiple delirium-producing narcotics given in ever-changing weekly dosages and combinations. The result of this harem-scarem, ego-tripping protocol was a return visit to the cardiac floor of the hospital.

Because the national nursing shortage gets worse every year, nursing errors are more and more common. Hospitals may call for overtime to compensate for the shortage, and others hire new and undertrained nurses to solve the problem. Many nurses admit that they struggle to stay awake while on duty, and others admit to falling asleep. Nurses do their best to deal with this broken system. Yet anyone who is overworked, has sleep deprivation, or is expected to perform tasks beyond their scope of ability may act carelessly and cause unwanted consequences.

Hospitals that don't have enough registered nurses can cause serious harm too. Research, published in the New England Journal of Medicine suggests a patient's risk of death increases by 2 percent per hospital shift when units are understaffed with registered nurses. And the risk of mortality increases with the number of shifts that are understaffed. When patients have three or more shifts with low staffing, the risk increases (2011).

Not only are registered nurses scarce; they are exhausted by patient overload, longer shifts, and rapid technological developments that call for new skills. And they are daunted by the ultimate headache—paper-work! One nurse told me the amount of paperwork was so paralyzing that she had little time to interact with patients. This was not why she went into nursing, and she regrettably had very little time to care for Mom's dire needs. So, lesser trained LPNs and assistants waded their way through Mom's complicated care.

The fallout from these conditions can be serious. According to The National Quality Forum, in the website article, *Safe Practices for Better Healthcare:*

- medical errors cause significant harm to patients in health care settings across the country;
- the Agency for Health Care Research and Quality (AHRQ) reported that preventable medical injuries are actually on the rise—by one percent a year;
- health care associated infections account for an estimated 1.7 million infections and 99,000 associated deaths each year;
- at least 1.5 million preventable drug events occur each year because of drug mix-ups and unintentional overdoses;
- eighteen types of medical errors account for 2.4 million extra hospital days and $9.3 billion in excess charges each year; and
- the harm can also be measured in heavy financial cost.

Preventable errors cost the United States $17–29 billion per year in health care expenses, lost worker productivity, lost income, and disability. Meanwhile, health care expenditures are growing at more than 7 percent per year, and patient safety is improving by only 1 percent. (2011)

The Joint Commission is the largest health care accrediting body in the United States. Their job is to accredit hospitals. They believe that public awareness is an important step in making things better. In March 2002, The Joint Commission launched a national campaign to urge patients to prevent errors by becoming active, involved, and informed participants. Research shows that patients who take part in decisions about their own care are more likely to get better faster. To help prevent health care mistakes, patients are urged to know the risks and to "Speak Up."

The following information on hospital risks is powerfully informative. Now you can understand the inner workings of a hospital—and how to navigate your way back home.

Medication Errors

Preventing Medical Errors, a report by the Institute of Medicine—advises Congress on health matters—and discloses, "on average, a hospital patient is subject to at least one medication error per day" (2006). It is frightening to know that medication mistakes in the hospital are not unusual. There is not a standardized way to measure the national or regional medication error rate. Most hospitals rely on voluntary reporting of errors, so it's easy to see that the public only hears about the "tip of the iceberg." Chances are you will never know if a medication error happens to you. Many times the hospital staff will not know unless you have a negative reaction to the error.

Mom survived a doozy. One morning, an extra talkative nurse came into the room, rambling on about her weekend. During her discourse, she confused two of the many IVs keeping Mom alive. She started an epinephrine drip that increases heart rate. At the time I didn't know epinephrine was a high-alert drug that carries a heightened risk of causing serious harm if used in error. While distracting herself with random chatter, the nurse set the pump to drip at the Vancomycin rate. Vancomycin is an antibiotic given in a different dose than an epinephrine dose. The yakking nurse left the room, unaware of her error.

Shortly after, my oldest daughter noticed an acute increase in Mom's heart rate and blood pressure. We quickly called for the nurses, and they checked all of the IVs. They stopped the epinephrine and summoned the guilty nurse. Another young nurse in the crowd attempted to console us by saying, "At least we caught it before the entire bag was administered." Mom was hanging on by a thread, and this event only caused additional trauma. I was livid, not only at the mistake, but by the attempt to brush it off by saying that it could have been worse.

The hospital filed an "incident report" and the "at fault" nurse was not allowed back in the room. Had she done it on purpose? Of course not. Was she upset that it happened? I know she was. Nevertheless, none of that negates that these things routinely happen, and someone other than the patient has to be observant.

What It Is

The five rules for the correct administration of medication are:

1. Right patient
2. Right drug
3. Right dose
4. Right route – by mouth, pill or liquid, intravenously, injection or inhaled
5. Right time

The five stages of the medication process are:

1. Ordering and prescribing
2. Transcribing and verifying
3. Dispensing and delivering
4. Administering
5. Monitoring and reporting

If these criteria are not met, there will be a consequence. Multiply this by the enormous amount of daily pills, injections, and IVs given by an itinerant team of doctors and nurses and you have a recipe for trouble. Sometimes the outcome can be mild, but often the mistake can seriously set you back and cause further complications, or worse, the result can be fatal.

How and Why It Happens

Two common causes of medication errors are illegible handwriting on the prescription and the use of abbreviations, especially concerning the dosage. A misplaced decimal point can be deadly. In an effort to prevent medication errors, The Joint Commission established a National Patient Safety Goal that specifies that certain abbreviations must not be used. For example, the initials OD for "once daily" could be mistaken for "Oculus Dexter," which stands for right eye. This could lead to an oral liquid medication administered to the right eye instead of taken by mouth once a day.

For interesting and educational reading about error-prone abbreviations, you may view the following resources:

- www.jointcommission.org/assets/1/18/Official_Do_Not_Use_ List_6_111.PDF
- www.ismp.org/tools/errorproneabbreviations.pdf

Another common cause of errors are drug names that look alike or sound alike, and products that have confusing drug labeling or similar packaging. Errors happen when a doctor interchanges two similar-sounding medications when writing an order, when the receiver misinterprets a written or verbal order, or when the order is entered incorrectly into the computer system.

A recent example from the Institute for Safe Medication Practices *Medication Safety Alert*: a heart transplant patient received Valtrex (valacyclovir) in error for ten days. The drug was supposed to be Valcyte (valganciclovir) and was chosen incorrectly from a computer selection screen (2009).

To download the list of confused drug names from the Institute for Safe Medication Practices: (www.ismp.org/tools/confuseddrugnames. pdf).

Errors often occur with medications that are not commonly used or when a patient no longer needs a particular medication. If the order to discontinue the drug does not transfer to the correct source, the patient may continue to take the unnecessary medication, sometimes with negative results.

Miscommunication between physicians, pharmacists, and nurses; verbal prescriptions and pharmacist error; and nurse fatigue can also negatively affect your safety. Medication errors usually involve the nursing staff. Nurses are the front line when it comes to administering and fulfilling doctors' orders, and may make mistakes because of sleep deprivation and exhaustion.

Additional risks for errors stem from lack of staff education, poor

systems and processes, and environmental issues such as noise, interruptions, patient overload, and staff shortages. Finally, those at highest
risk for error are uneducated patients who do not ask questions, do not
know what medications they are taking, and blindly rely on the hospital
staff to do their jobs correctly.

What to Look For

- A change in regime—too few pills as usual, more pills than
  usual, different colored or sized pills, missed dosages, double
  dosages, or medication administered at a different time of day
  are signs that someone might have made an error.
- An unusual reaction including a rash, headache, swelling, dizziness, or trouble breathing could indicate an incorrect dose or a
  wrong medication.
- A nurse or hospital staff member that tends to you longer than
  eight hours each day may be working a double shift or more
  and might be prone to making errors.
- If you move rooms, have a roommate, or if a patient down
  the hall has a similar name—you may run the risk of receiving
  someone else's medication.
- Anything that doesn't seem or feel right to you is a potential
  sign of trouble.

How to Protect Yourself

Upon admission to the hospital, your doctor or nurse will record the
names and dosages of all your current medications and any over the
counter drugs, vitamins, and herbal supplements. Usually there is no
need to bring your medicines from home to the hospital. You should
get what you need throughout your hospital stay. Explain any allergies,
previous adverse drug reactions, or bad experiences with anesthesia you
have had.

If you have drug allergies, you will get a separate allergy bracelet
upon admission. Check the wristband for accuracy. Hospital staff
should verify the band each time they give you a drug, perform a diagnostic test, or take a blood sample. If they don't, advise them of your

name and any other information they might need. Always check the IV fluids to be sure that they are marked with your correct name as well as the correct drug and dose as ordered by the doctor.

As an informed patient or advocate, you need to understand all medications—the names, dosages, frequency, what they are for, any potential food or drug interactions, and possible side effects. Be on the lookout for any medications that look alike or have names that sound alike. Speak up if you don't get medication when you should; this is the most common of drug errors.

High-alert medications carry a heightened risk because they can cause considerable harm when used in error. The FDA uses a black box warning system with the highest caution requirements to alert consumers to drugs with serious adverse risks, namely severe injury or death. The common drugs, Ritalin and Celebrex, estrogen-containing contraceptives, the antibiotics Cipro and Levaquin, and most antidepressants carry black box warnings. Black box drugs are tricky in that they can be dosage form specific, meaning the danger can vary depending how the medication is administered (e.g., orally, intravenously, or inhaled). Find out if you are taking any high alert medications.

For additional information on high alert medications, see the following online resources:

- Institute for Safe Medication Practices (www.ismp.org/tools/highalertmedications.pdf)
- BlackBoxRx.com (http://blackboxrx.com)

Medications may be listed by their trade names or their generic names, and this can get confusing. Ask your doctor and nurses if you are unsure. Keep both names written in your safety log. Some may call a drug by the generic name and others may use the trade name. If you know both, you will be safe.

The nurses use a *medication administration record sheet* called MARS. This is a daily list of medications and dosages that indicate which drugs to administer to you throughout the day. If the doctor changes or discontinues a particular drug, that change is reflected on the next day's MARS. You or your advocate can ask for these forms each morning so you can observe and track the continuity of medications. Store your daily MARS in a folder. Remember to take current copies of these sheets with you if you transfer to a different floor or location to ensure continuity of medication during transfer.

When prescribed new medications, ask your doctors to explain their purposes and any potential side effects. Make sure that any new medications do not conflict with your current medications or with any allergies you may have. It will also be helpful for you to record your medication names and dosages and any negative reactions you may have had.

If you don't feel comfortable taking something you don't recognize, speak up. You have every right to refuse a medication that you feel might be given to you in error. I admired one family on Mom's floor. They insisted the medications be brought to the room in their initial packaging from the pharmacy. Ask your nurses not to open the pill wrappers before they bring them to you. This is just another way to protect yourself and your loved ones.

Your vigilance doesn't end when your hospital stay is over. Understand which drugs you are supposed to take when you are discharged. Ask about the drugs you have at home and if you should continue to take them. Keep a current list of drugs and dosages with you at all times in case you go to an urgent care, emergency room, or another doctor. In the end, you and your advocate are the best weapons against medication errors.

Infection

In a *Hand Hygiene* brochure created by The Centers for Disease Control and Prevention, an estimated 2 million patients acquire an infection in the hospital every year. Nearly one in twenty patients is affected, totaling 100,000 deaths per year. This places hospital-acquired infections (HAIs) as the fourth leading cause of death in the United States (2011). Many reasons contribute to this problem, including increasing rates of antibiotic resistance; new, complex, and invasive medical technology; a shortage of qualified nurses; an increasing elderly patient population and dirty hands.

The risk of serious complications because of HAIs is greater for patients requiring intensive care. Most of these infections are preventable through simple methods including hand washing and the early removal of catheters and central lines. The good news is that as a patient or an advocate, you have a real ability to reduce your chances of acquiring an infection by making infection control your top concern.

What It Is

Nosocomial is the medical term for hospital-acquired or health care-associated infection. I heard a nurse use this word as she spoke to an aide while reviewing Mom's chart. I thought it was a rare disease. When I looked it up and learned the meaning, I asked the nurse, "Exactly what hospital-acquired infection does Mom have?" She responded, "Are you a nurse?" No—just an educated consumer.

Dangerous germs spread both directly and indirectly. Because doctors and nurses travel from patient to patient, the staff is usually responsible for direct contamination. Your doctors and nurses interact with you hundreds of times each day. They examine you, administer drugs, adjust your bed, or bathe you. If they do not wash their hands each time they enter your room, they physically transfer infectious microorganisms all over you and your room. Contaminated lab coats and neckties also contribute to hospital- acquired infections. Recently, I viewed a webinar on the website, *Infection Control Today*, (www.infectioncontroltoday. com) and learned of a study that asked 140 doctors how often they washed their lab coats. One third responded once per week. Another third responded every two weeks and the last third admitted to once per month. In the same study, some residents declared they never washed their lab coat (2011). Because organisms can survive on fabric for 90 days, these are scary facts.

Nasty pathogens can spread indirectly by way of contaminated dressings; intravenous devices, needles and flushes; stethoscopes; blood pressure cuffs; telemetry units; hospital gowns, and gloves. Invasive catheters, intubation tubes, and surgical drains also provide easy routes for infection. Blood transfusions, antibiotic regimes, and cancer therapy leave the body in a susceptible state.

During a hospital stay, you are in a weakened condition. This predisposition allows germs to take hold and multiply quickly. The combination of seriously ill patients, the overuse use of antibiotics, and cross-contamination result in infections whose pathogens many times do not leave the body, even months after hospital discharge. This makes you and the community at large susceptible to further problems.

Hospital-acquired infections come by many names and varieties. Here are a few of the most common (which I explain later):

- methicillin resistant *Staphylococcus aureus* (MRSA)
- clostridium difficile (C diff)
- central line associated bloodstream infections (CLABSI)
- hospital-acquired pneumonia (HAP)
- ventilator associated pneumonia (VAP)
- klebsiella
- catheter associated urinary tract infection (CAUTI)
- infections due to antibiotic resistant super bugs such as vancomycin-resistant enterococcus (VRE)
- surgical site infection (SSI), IV site infection, injection site infection

How and Why it Happens

Hand hygiene is the most important component in the prevention of hospital-acquired infections. From an article, *Hospital infection is the next asbestos,* by the Committee to Reduce Infection Deaths, at least half of hospital infections are preventable if caregivers clean their hands immediately before touching patients. Doctors are the main culprits; they break this elementary tenet 52 percent of the time, on average and intensive care units showed that hand washing occurred only one quarter of the essential times (2011).

Hospitals have training sessions devoted to hand washing. Signs are posted throughout the floors, reminding people to wash their hands. Sinks, soaps, paper towels, and antibacterial gel pumps are everywhere. Hand washing doesn't cost anything, yet hospital-acquired infections cost the country billions of dollars annually. The average price of treating an infection with MRSA, a staph bacteria resistant to many antibiotics, is close to $50,000. This is an expensive problem, both monetarily and riskwise, yet part of the solution is so basic and cheap.

In addition to hand washing, gloves play an important part in infection control and are used to protect both the caregiver and the patient. Gloves act as a barrier to protect the caregiver from contamination when touching blood, body fluids, and open wounds. Gloves also prevent transmission of germs from the caregiver to the patient. Finally, gloves lessen the chance of the caregiver transmitting germs from one patient to another.

The concept of gloves is rudimentary, yet on many occasions during Mom's hospital stay, I observed serious mismanagement of glove use. One morning the entire wound team arrived to change the dressing on Mom's bedsore. As they moved about, one of the nurses knocked my water bottle on the floor. In the midst of cleaning the open sore, she paused, reached down with her gloved hand, picked up my bottle, and placed it back on the table. Then she resumed with the dressing change. Not only did she contaminate my bottle, she also contaminated her glove with the germs from my bottle and the germs the bottle picked up from the floor. When I mentioned this to her, she apologized, took off the gloves and grabbed a new pair. Ideally, she should have washed her hands before putting on the new gloves, as she had contaminated her hands when she took off the old gloves.

This incident shows how improper hand and glove hygiene creates an infection control hazard. Had I not seen this, I would have picked up my water bottle to take a drink, not knowing that bloody bedsore gloves had contaminated my supposed refreshment. After that experience, I wiped the entire room with antibacterial wipes at least twice each day.

Sanitizing the surfaces in your hospital room is a simple way to break the infection cycle. Germs can survive on surfaces for extended periods. Frequently touched surfaces or disease transfer points include bed rails, call buttons, television remotes, over-the-bed trays, chairs, telephones, door handles, light switches, intravenous poles, soap and towel dispensers, sinks, toilets, grab bars, counters, and tabletops. These surfaces are known to be contaminated with staphylococcus and methicillin-resistant *Staphylococcus aureus* (MRSA)—some of the most potent strains of antibiotic-resistant bacteria—and other pathogens. Objects that are used most often and are closest to your bed have the highest levels of bacteria. These surfaces are prime ways you, the hospital staff, and your visitors can spread bacteria.

Housekeepers and transporters are among the most mobile hospital personnel. Because of this, they may spread hospital infections. On a recent hospital visit, I watched a transporter enter a patient's room across the hallway. He did not wash or sanitize his hands. He touched the patient, the bed, and the gurney as he assisted with the transfer. I left Mom's room and walked behind him as I headed to the cafeteria. I stopped to watch him drop the patient off at the X-ray department. He received a message on his pager and turned around to pick up another patient. Throughout this transfer, he did not clean his hands. I wondered, "Are the sheets and pillowcases replaced with clean ones?" "Does someone sanitize the bed rails?" "Does the transporter ever wash his hands?" If this cycle continues, can you imagine how much cross-contamination takes place?

MRSA

Methicillin resistant *Staphylococcus Aureus* (MRSA) is a form of staph infection resistant to some antibiotics. Many people are colonized with MRSA, meaning the bacteria is present in their bodies but does not cause symptoms or problems. When someone is infected, the bacterium actually invades the body and causes signs of illness. A break in the skin caused by anything—a simple cut, an IV or catheter site, a wound, or a surgical site—is an entry point that can lead to an infection. If the infection reaches the bloodstream, the problem becomes more serious.

Because MRSA can live on the skin, those who unknowingly carry the bacteria can leave it on hard surfaces including wheelchairs, stethoscopes, blood pressure cuffs, door handles, and any other area they touch. It spreads easily and is remarkably indifferent to antibiotics, making MRSA one of the deadliest of hospital infections. This makes me fear the wheelchairs found at most hospital entrance doors, graciously awaiting patients who need ambulatory help. How many people who are colonized with MRSA or who have active infections use these chairs? The public also has free access to them, making wheelchairs high-touch, infection-carrying vehicles. Many studies also show that ambulances and rescue vehicles are contaminated with MRSA in addition to other contagious pathogens.

Clothing is another common carrier for infections, especially MRSA. When doctors and nurses lean over a patient who has MRSA, their clothing and uniforms pick up bacteria allowing transfer to other patients. MRSA has an extensive life, with the ability to linger on clothing and surfaces long after a hospital room is unoccupied. The bacterium remains on floors, beds, tables, and other surfaces from previous infected patients. This demonstrates how virulent this infection is and why you need to do everything you can to avoid it. Hospitals sometimes implement a preadmission nasal swab screening of all surgical patients to detect those with MRSA. This procedure has its proponents and opponents, so you may want to ask your doctor or hospital what precautions they take to prevent MRSA.

C DIFF

Another rampant infection, clostridium difficile associated disease (CDAD) —better known as C diff—is a bacterium that causes diarrhea or colitis and develops from prolonged use of antibiotics during a hospital stay. Certain people naturally carry C diff in their bodies. Healthy stomach flora prevents symptoms. The use of antibiotics can kill all of the bacteria in the gut, both good and bad. This allows C diff to multiply and flourish. Severe, watery diarrhea and inflammation of the colon develops, and contamination usually from hands to the mouth causes a rapid and out-of-control spread of this lethal bacterium.

C diff produces spores transmitted through feces that survive for months. Because the spores can travel through the air, an infectious film of C diff spores can live on every surface of your room, especially in bathrooms. A study in the Journal of Hospital Infection titled *National Clostridium difficile Standards Group: Report to the Department of Health*, shows that one-third of blood pressure cuffs used from room to room carry C diff spores on the inside of the cuff (2004). Because C diff usually spreads from hand to mouth, good hygiene and housekeeping are mandatory. You can become infected by touching contaminated surfaces and then touching your nose or mouth or you can contaminate your food. C diff spores are not eradicated by hand gels and sanitizers. Soap, water, and correct hand-washing techniques, along with reduced antibiotic treatments, are best practices to reduce the presence of C diff. To disinfect surfaces, use bleach at a 1:10 dilution in water. The Cleveland Veterans Affair Medical Center evaluated an infection prevention program that concluded:

> A 1:10 bleach (DISPATCH®) solution for routine disinfection of high-touch surfaces found reduced C diff rates by 67 percent. They also assessed six high-touch surfaces in rooms with Vancomycin-resistant Enterococcus (VRE)—before cleaning and after typical cleaning and after 1:10 bleach disinfection to determine if including 1:10 bleach for surface disinfection could reduce contamination of these surfaces. Using 1:10 bleach (DISPATCH®) solution for routine disinfection of high-touch surfaces reduced positive VRE detection rates by 100%. The program was sustained for four months with results maintained (2007).

CLABSI

Central line-associated bloodstream infections (CLABSIs) result in thousands of deaths each year and billions of dollars in added costs to the U.S. health care system, yet these infections are preventable. A central line is a tube placed in a large vein to deliver drugs and nutrition. If the line is inserted incorrectly or not kept clean, it becomes a direct route for germs to enter the body and can cause serious bloodstream infections. A central line becomes contaminated when the skin site harbors a germ like staph or candida or when a hand or glove touching the line is contaminated. Intensive care patients are at a high risk of developing CLABSI because of the need for multiple catheters, which are often inserted under emergency situations and stay intact for long periods.

HAP and VAP

Hospital-acquired pneumonia (HAP) is any pneumonia or infection of the lungs contracted between two to three days after admission to the hospital. It is the second most common HAI after urinary tract infections. Of all the HAIs, HAP is the number one cause of death, and it is the primary cause of death in intensive care units. Patients who use any mechanical ventilation or heavy antibiotics; older adults; and patients with swallowing difficulties or abdominal surgery are at extra risk for HAP.

In an article from the American Society of Microbiology, called *Ventilator-Associated Pneumonia: Diagnosis, Treatment, and Prevention*: "Patients in the intensive care unit (ICU) are at risk for dying not only from their critical illness but also from secondary processes such as nosocomial infection. Pneumonia is the second most common nosocomial infection in critically ill patients, affecting 27% of all critically ill patients. Eighty-six percent of nosocomial pneumonias are associated with mechanical ventilation and are termed ventilator-associated pneumonia (VAP)" (2006).

VAP is a pneumonia that develops more than forty-eight hours after endotracheal intubation or forty-eight hours of extubation or removal. VAP occurs when bacteria invades the respiratory tract and lungs and is further compromised by breathing tubes. The Center for Disease Control's National Nosocomial Infection Surveillance System reports that patients receiving continuous mechanical ventilation have up to twenty-one times the risk of developing hospital-acquired pneumonia compared with patients who do not receive mechanical ventilation (2003).

Klebsiella

Klebsiella is a bacterium from the Enterobacteriaceae family that can cause many kinds of hospital-acquired infections, including pneumonia, bloodstream infections, wound or surgical site infections, and meningitis. The bacteria can live in the human intestines where they do not cause disease. Sick patients in health care settings, who receive treatment for other conditions often develop *Klebsiella* infections. Patients who need ventilators (breathing machines) or intravenous catheters and patients who take long courses of certain antibiotics are most at risk for *Klebsiella* infections. The bacteria spread through person-to-person contact or through contamination of the environment, making hand hygiene imperative. The bacteria do not spread through the air. *Klebsiella* bacteria are highly resistant to antibiotics and are difficult to treat, making prevention the rule.

CAUTI

Catheter-associated urinary tract infections (CAUTIs) develop when bacteria enters the urinary tract through the urinary catheter. CAUTIs account for an astounding 80 percent of HAIs in hospitals. More than 30,000 patients die in the hospital from bloodstream infections they get from catheters. According to an excerpt taken from a Center for Disease Control's Healthcare Infection Control Practices Advisory Committee document titled *Guideline for Prevention of Catheter-Associated Urinary Tract Infections:*

> Urinary tract infections are the most common type of health-care-associated infection. Virtually all healthcare-associated urinary tract infections are caused by instrumentation of the urinary tract. Catheter-associated urinary tract infection has been associated with increased morbidity, mortality, hospital cost and length of stay. In addition, bacteria commonly lead to unnecessary antimicrobial use, and urinary drainage systems are often reservoirs for multidrug-resistant bacteria and a source of transmission to other patients. (2009)

Many times, catheters remain longer than needed, which creates breeding grounds for infections. Mom had a urine catheter for four months. The doctors wanted to remove it for infection reasons. However, she had a large stage four pressure sore located in an area that could easily get soaked with urine if the nurses did not respond quickly to a bedpan call—and the nursing staff was notorious for responding to call buttons in slow motion. When I expressed these concerns to the staff, no one offered to make her bathroom calls a priority; so, the catheter remained, and we played roulette with CAUTI for months.

VRE

Vancomycin-resistant enterococci (VRE) are bacteria normally present in the human intestines, the female genital tract and in the environment. These bacteria can sometimes cause infections of the urinary tract, the bloodstream or wounds associated with catheters or surgical procedures. Vancomycin is an antibiotic used to treat drug-resistant infections caused by these bacteria. Enterococci have become resistant to Vancomycin and therefore called vancomycin-resistant enterococci. Most VRE infections take place in hospitals. Usually VRE infections respond to antibiotics other than vancomycin. For patients who have VRE infections in their bladder and have urinary catheters, removal of the catheter when it is no longer needed helps get rid of the infection. As with other hospital-acquired infections, VRE spreads from person to person by hand and surface contamination. Wash hands frequently, use alcohol based hand sanitizers and wear gloves. VRE does not spread through the air by sneezing or coughing.

Surgical site infection, IV site infection, injection site infection

A surgical site infection (SSI) is an infection that develops after surgery in the part of the body or at the site where the surgery took place. Common symptoms of a surgical site infection are redness and pain around the area where you had surgery, drainage of cloudy fluid from your surgical wound and fever. Most surgical site infections are treated with antibiotics or sometimes, another surgery. An IV site or injection site can also become infected. Improper use of syringe's and liquid medications administered using a needle may not only cause an infection, but possibly a secondary disease. A warning from the Centers for Disease Control and Prevention:

> Patients need to be aware of a very serious threat to their health - the reuse of needles or syringes, and the misuse of medication vials. Your healthcare providers should **never reuse a needle or syringe** from one patient to another or to withdraw medicine from a vial. Both needle and syringe must be discarded after each use. It is not safe to change the needle and reuse the syringe as this practice can transmit disease.

> A single-use vial is a bottle of liquid medication given to a patient through a needle and syringe. Single-use vials contain only one dose of medication used once for one patient, using a clean needle and clean syringe. A multi-dose vial is a bottle of

liquid medication that contains more than one dose of medication often used by diabetic patients or for vaccinations. A
new, clean needle and clean syringe should be used to access the
medication in a multi-dose vial. Reuse of needles or syringes to
access medication can result in contamination of the medicine
with germs that can spread to others when the medicine is used
again. Reusing a needle or syringe puts patients in danger of
contracting Hepatitis C, Hepatitis B and possibly HIV. (2011)

Make sure your health care providers enforce the rule: 1 Needle + 1
Syringe + 1 Time = 0 Infections.

What to Look For

Certain issues may leave you vulnerable to an infection. Risk factors
that may increase your chance of acquiring an infection during a hospital
stay include:

- a long hospital stay, multiple hospitalizations or multiple invasive procedures
- patient age of sixty-five or older
- wounds, severe disease or critically ill
- repeated antibiotic therapy or vancomycin use
- ICU patients or patients in cancer or transplant units
- an abdominal or cardiothoracic surgical procedure
- a urinary or central venous catheter or use of a ventilator
- chronic kidney disease
- low nurse-to-patient ratio
- ambulance transporters and vehicle equipment
- improper hand-washing and glove use

Before you go to the hospital, inquire about the hospital's infection
safety and error rate and ask to meet the person who manages it. A
rating above 3 percent is not acceptable. Choose a primary care doctor
with admitting privileges at the cleanest hospital and let your doctor
know you will be diligent about monitoring infection possibilities.

The Consumer Reports website lists hospital ratings by state at www. consumerreports.org/health/doctors-hospitals/hospital-ratings.htm.

How to Protect Yourself

For Patients and Their Advocates

Hand-washing and surface sanitation go a long way to prevent many hospital-acquired infections. It is easy to do, does not cost anything, and could very well save your life. Make infection control your goal. Speak up if others do not share your enthusiasm for this simple infection remedy. Remember, you are not in the hospital to make friends with the hospital staff. Your goal is to get out alive. Who cares if people think you're cuckoo for insisting they wash their hands? For the most part, the staff will admire you for standing up for your right to stay safe. Ask everyone who comes into your room to wash their hands.

You can set an example for staff and visitors by following your own rules: wash your hands many times throughout the day, especially before you eat and before and after using the toilet or bedpan. Also, your nose and throat may be colonized with MRSA, so after you blow your nose, dispose of the tissue with care, wash your hands, and use antibacterial gel. Keep a bottle of antibacterial gel next to your hospital bed. Make sure everyone uses it before touching you.

Ask if the prior patient occupying your room had MRSA or C diff. If the answer is yes, request another room. Wipe, wipe, wipe. Either you or your advocate must wipe everything in the room with disinfectant. Wear gloves when you clean to avoid contaminating your hands. Use one wipe for each surface to prevent cross-contamination from surface to surface and discard after use. Do not re-use a wipe.

C diff bacteria or spores are ingested by mouth, so routinely clean your hands throughout the day, especially before meals. I even wash hospital silverware before use. Clean your bed tray with disinfectant before and after your meal tray is delivered

Dry or cracked skin can be an entry point for MRSA. Keep hand lotion nearby and use it often. Do not touch wounds, dressings, bandages, or catheters because the bacteria on your hands can cause infection.

I recently met a woman from Rhode Island who created a practical and much-needed solution to help with hand hygiene. She suffered through a hospital nightmare with a parent and because of this chose to make positive changes in patient outcomes.

Bob Stegeman entered the hospital for neck surgery and suffered many medical complications over the six months that followed. His daughter, Pat Mastors, was at his bedside when he died in the hospital of complications from the hospital-acquired infection C diff. The anxiety and helplessness, Pat and her family felt during this time was overwhelming.

When asked about her ordeal, Pat said, "Within weeks Dad went from a stubbornly independent man who still fixed his car and mowed his own lawn to a frail, dependent shell of himself. His caregivers rotated constantly, and his room switched a dozen times. It was frustrating that on top of his medical challenges, we were always posting notes and reminding caregivers about Dad's hearing problem (during his first days in the hospital, water spilled on his hearing aids and ruined them). It was even more frustrating for my father, and eventually he gave up trying to communicate. Every time I left Dad's hospital room, I wondered if he would be able to find his things or if people would remember to speak loudly when they talked to him. The experience ate away at his health and his dignity."

This experience led Pat to improve safety, dignity, and autonomy for all hospital patients. She started an informational website to inform other families about infection risk and prevention strategies, worked through her state legislature to pass new patient safety laws, and began to actively collaborate with other patient advocates around the country. However, some basic questions still troubled her.

Because good hand hygiene is so important to infection prevention, how are immobilized patients supposed to clean their hands? (Hand sanitizer is typically bolted to the wall, out of reach.) When she learned of the University of Arizona's research showing the most germ-laden item in the hospital room is the TV remote, she wondered if the remote control could be covered the same way gloves cover hands. When her father's hearing aids were ruined in the hospital, she questioned why there hadn't been a protected, dedicated place for the patient to put personal items. (She later learned that hearing aids and dentures are often left on dinner trays and tossed in the trash.) Finally, she thought there should be a way to advise every caregiver "at a glance" that a patient was hard of hearing or had a special need.

Using her twenty years of experience as a news and medical reporter, she started a research process, asking patients, families, caregivers, and hospital administrators to share their insights and "wish lists." With that, she invented the Patient Pod, a heavy-duty vinyl personal storage system coupled to a unique, swiveling attachment clamp. It clamps to the bed rail and keeps personal items within reach. The front of the Patient Pod has space for a personal photo and identification and offers a special clip to post messages, questions, or reminders. The Pod comes prepackaged with hand sanitizer and wipes, custom covers for the TV remote, a notepad and pen, and essential tips on how to partner with caregivers to guard against infection. It's an ingenious yet simple solution worth adding to your safety tools.

You can also place a sign or poster above your bed that says, "Please wash your hands before touching me." If you are unable to speak or asleep, your advocate can simply point to the sign when a health care provider enters the room. The clip on the Patient Pod is also a perfect place to post the reminder. It is not rude or weird to ask everyone to wash their hands or to be concerned about bacteria on stethoscopes or blood pressure cuffs. You can request dedicated equipment, especially a blood pressure cuff, a wheelchair if needed, a pulse oximeter, and other necessary items. If you can't have your own equipment, use an antibacterial body wipe to clean your skin after a potential infectious encounter. Keep a large container of antibacterial wipes and a roll of paper towels and a spray bottle of bleach water (1:10 bleach concentration) in your room at all times. I used to keep mine on the windowsill behind the curtains. Either you or your advocate should wipe every surface in the room both in the morning and at night. Pay extra attention to frequently touched areas and the bathroom.

Telemetry monitors are also vehicles that spread bacteria and infections. These monitors supervise heart rhythm changes, respiration and oxygen saturation. You'll know you are on a telemetry-monitored floor if your nurse attaches ECG leads to your chest and back. The leads are circular, about the size of a half dollar and stick to your skin with an adhesive. Next, a transmitter—similar to a transistor radio—is attached to the leads by way of wires. Your hospital gown may have a pocket to hold the transmitter, or you may carry it around your neck in a soft pouch-like purse. Antennas located in the hospital allow your information to transfer to receivers at the main monitoring station where trained nurses or technicians keep watch. Cross-contamination of the lead wires and the telemetry unit are an infection concern. A telemetry transmitter can be contaminated by a patient's body fluids, wound drainage or unwashed hands allowing infections to spread from one patient to another. The ECG lead wires are difficult to clean, if they are cleaned at all. The wires and unit often come in direct contact with the skin on a patient's back, stomach, trunk and arms for long periods. Hospital protocol does not always make clear who is responsible for cleaning medical equipment between patients. Or those assigned to clean may forget or be lazy. The morning mom was discharged from the telemetry unit, a nurse removed the lead wires, pulled the transmitter out of mom's hospital gown pocket and placed it on her bed tray, needlessly contaminating that surface. Moments later, another nurse ran it, grabbed the transmitter from the table and said, "I need this for room 3031." Off she went to the room across the hall. No gloves—no disinfecting—no concern. Mr. 3031 now enjoyed a month's worth of mom's bacteria, delivered directly to his chest and back. Disposable ECG leads and telemetry pouches do exist. Tell your doctor or nurse to assign a dedicated disposable ECG lead package and telemetry pouch for your use throughout your stay. If they do not have disposable ones, ask for non-used or freshly sanitized equipment.

Nurses aren't the only ones who dash in and out of your room. The housekeeping staff stops by each day to clean and empty the trash. Because they travel from room to room, they are frontrunners for spreading infections. Housekeeping personnel have a high turnover rate. Therefore, many housekeepers are new and not thoroughly trained or experienced in infection control. They should put on a new pair of gloves when they enter your room. Share your concern about infection and ask them to clean all surfaces with a disinfectant. Make sure they use a brand new cleaning cloth or towel for each area of your room. One afternoon, I watched a hospital housekeeper clean Mom's bed tray with the same cloth she used in the bathroom. How about C diff with your next meal? Ask for a new mop head too.

On my last visit to the hospital, I asked about the logic in smearing blood, body fluids, and bacteria from room to room in the name of floor cleaning. I learned a lot about floor mopping procedures. Hospital floors are mopped daily with heavy-duty chemicals and the traditional loop mop, bucket and wringer—or with the newer microfiber mops. With loop mops, the water is supposed to be changed every two to three rooms and the mop head washed at the end of the shift. The only way this sounds good to me is if I am the first room of the day. The microfiber mop resembles a Swiffer and has removable cloths. Each room is supposed to be double cleaned with both sides of the cloth. The microfiber mopping system eliminates cross-contamination from room to room because clean cloths are used in every room. The only way to be sure this actually happens is to watch the housekeeper as he or she enters your room. If in doubt, ask for a new cloth. To make it easy for housekeeping to clean all areas, keep personal items to a minimum and off the floor. If you notice negligence when it comes to mopping, cleaning and infection control, say something. Sub-optimal cleaning practices are simply not acceptable.

The staff should not enter your room wearing a disposable gown or mask used in a previous room. If C diff and MRSA are present on your floor, insist that everyone wear a brand new gown as they enter your room. Mom had three precarious encounters with C diff and was on "contact precaution." Boxes of disposable gowns and masks graced her entrance door. Every time the staff came in, they put on a new gown and discarded it in the trash before they left. However, none of this is worth-while if glove procedures are ignored. Wearing gloves does not replace the need for hand washing. Gloves may have small tears or other openings not visible to the eye. Doctors and nurses are supposed to wash their hands before putting on gloves. Gloves are removed by pulling them off inside out. Touching the gloves with bare skin should be avoided, and hands washed again in case they are contaminated during glove removal.

It is also important not to contaminate your bed. Make sure your pillowcase is clean. If it falls on the floor or becomes dirty, request a new one. Now that you understand the floor washing procedure, you see

why it is unsafe to use anything that touches the floor. You especially do
not want to go barefoot anywhere in a hospital. It's a good practice to
keep dedicated pairs of socks or footies—one for your bed and one for
the floor. The hospital will supply these if you need extras. Do not allow
visitors to sit on your bed or put purses or other such items on your bed.

For surgery patients, another way to avoid infections is to use an
antibiotic nasal swab. A nasal ointment called mupirocin (Bactroban)
used before surgery reduces the rate of hospital-acquired staph infections among patients who are carriers. However, the overuse of powerful
broad-spectrum antibiotics breeds drug-resistant germs. Always show
your concern for antibiotics and stay informed. Inquire about probiotics
to help counteract the negative effects of antibiotics. Before surgery, you
may be asked to bathe or shower with chlorhexidine soap to help mitigate a surgical site infection.

The following precautions can help prevent catheter associated
urinary tract infections: If you are still using a urine catheter forty-eight
hours after surgery, find out when it will be removed. The risk of infection increases when the urinary catheter is left in place for more than
two or three days. If you feel urinary discomfort or pain, ask your nurse
to check for clogs. Make certain the catheter and bag receive daily care
and maintenance. Clean your hands and insist all health care providers
scrub their hands before and after touching the catheter. When a caregiver changes the catheter, make sure the tubing is not exposed to your
bed sheets or anything else that may harbor bacteria. Position the urine
bag below the level of the bladder, and do not pull o twist the catheter
tubing.

To prevent ventilator-acquired pneumonia, ask if you need a prophy-
lactic antibiotic an hour before the surgical incision. If shaving of the
surgical site is suggested, ask if clipping or a depilatory can be used.
Shaving causes small nicks in the skin, which could contribute to potential surgical site infections. Additional prevention measures include
elevating the head of your bed at a 30 to 45° angle. If you are the advocate, make sure your patient is not in a constant state of sedation. A
daily interruption of sedation leads to reduced cases of VAP. Also, brush
the patient's teeth. Oral infections can spread to the lungs. Each day, ask

about any chest X-ray or sputum culture results. Keep an eye out for fevers that might indicate an infection in the lungs.

Personal hygiene items can also contribute to the spread of infection. Bring clean or new personal items including a toothbrush and toothpaste, combs, and shaving items, and throw them away when discharged. Pack only freshly laundered clothes for use in the hospital.

Keep a few clean paper towels or plastic baggies in your purse or pocket. Use them to cover your hands when opening hospital doors, for wheelchair handles, elevator buttons, or any other public surface. Toss when through, do not reuse them. Bring your own pen. How many sick patients sign their hospital admission forms with the same pen? Start you hospital stay by making infection control your goal.

For Advocates and Visitors

To keep your patient as safe as possible, scrub your hands before entering and leaving the room. Do not sit on the bed or touch any equipment. If you are sick or feeling ill, it's best to stay home. If you sneeze, cough, or wipe your nose during your visit, dispose of the tissue carefully and wash your hands, then use antibacterial gel. Use the public restroom instead of the patient's bathroom, and bring disinfectant with you for toilet handles, sink knobs, and doorknobs. Scrub your hands before and after using the restroom.

Help your patient with infection control by keeping the room clean and wiping all surfaces with disinfectant. He or she may not feel well enough to do this. For your protection, wipe your chair with disinfectant wipes before you sit in case bacteria lives on the chair. Wipe it down again before you leave to protect the patient in the event you carried germs on your clothing.

Keep your purse and personal belongings off the floor and off the patient's bed. I always wiped the bottom of my purse with antiseptic wipes as I left the hospital to avoid carrying bacteria to my car and home. Once home, I wiped my shoes with disinfectant and changed clothes immediately. After a long day in a germ-filled hospital, I could not imagine sitting on my couch with bacteria on my clothes.

Take care of yourself by paying attention to infection opportunities. Waiting room magazines, TV remotes, elevator buttons, doorknobs, restrooms, fresh fruits and vegetables from the cafeteria, or any other raw food handled by several people are potential sources of bacteria. Drink lots of water, eat healthy foods (preferably packed from home), and take supplements and probiotics.

The opportunity to acquire an infection in the hospital is huge. Germs and bacteria are everywhere. They float in the air, live on your clothes and hands, and reside on everything in sight. The consequences of a hospital-acquired infection are grave, yet prevention is simple. Be a germaphobe. Be a clean freak.

Adverse Drug Reactions and Side Effects

Sometimes medicine causes more harm than it does good. Millions of patients have in-hospital adverse drug reactions (ADRs) to prescribed medicine because of the inherent toxicity of the drugs rather than to allergic reactions. As more drugs become available, the number of adverse drug reactions is likely to increase. Drugs are a business, and the culprits are many:

- pharmaceutical companies with their expensive television and print advertising campaigns and dedicated drug representatives who romance doctors with free samples
- some pharmacists who sell doctors' prescribing lists or who work for drug companies
- pharmacy organizations, the American Pharmaceutical Association and others who fight to prevent the Food and Drug Administration (FDA) from requiring the inclusion of accurate patient information with each filled prescription
- the FDA, who is not in your corner but instead chooses to side with the drug industry by approving dangerous drugs prematurely and not monitoring drug ads
- some physicians who choose to learn about drugs and their potential side effects from the drug companies or drug-company-sponsored research
- you the patient, who blindly wants to believe that the drug companies, government, pharmacists, and doctors make decisions to benefit you and not them

Many of the experts hired to advise the government on the safety and effectiveness of medicine have financial relationships with the pharmaceutical companies that will be helped or hurt by their decisions. These experts are hired to advise the FDA on which medicines should be approved for sale, what the warning labels should say, and how studies of drugs should be designed. The experts are supposed to be independent, yet many times have a direct financial interest in the drug or topic they evaluate. These conflicts include helping a pharmaceutical company develop a medicine and then serving on an FDA advisory committee to judge the drug. Many FDA officials were previously employed by major drug companies before joining the FDA and conversely, upon leaving the FDA, take executive jobs in pharmaceutical companies.

The paper, *Creating Demand for Prescription Drugs: A Content Analysis of Television Direct-to-Consumer Advertising,* from the Annals of Family Medicine, Inc., states:

> The United States and New Zealand are the only developed countries that permit direct-to-consumer advertising of prescription drugs. Average American television viewers see up to 16 hours of prescription drug advertisements per year, far exceeding the average time spent with a primary care physician. Despite claims that ads serve an educational purpose, they provide limited information about the causes of a disease or who may be at risk; they show characters that have lost control over their social, emotional, or physical lives without the medication; and they minimize the value of health promotion through lifestyle changes. The ads have limited educational value and may oversell the benefits of drugs in ways that might conflict with promoting population health. (2007)

I remember the first time I watched the energy drink campaign introducing the 2:30 Feeling. At first, I felt out of the loop. Why haven't I experienced the 2:30 feeling? Then I got irritated to see how a business, in an attempt to make a profit, creates a debatable ailment that does not need treatment. Never mind that energy drinks are dangerous. If there is a 2:30 feeling, how about making a simple and safe lifestyle change by eating a handful of almonds and an apple? Oh, that's right. Where's the money in that?

What It Is

An adverse drug reaction (ADR) is an unintended and undesired effect that causes harm, and is associated with the use of medications given at a normal dosage. ADRs may occur following one dose or from prolonged administration of a drug, or they can result from the combination of two or more drugs. A side effect is a nearly unavoidable and predictable secondary effect of a drug. The intensity of the side effect depends on the dosage size.

Both ADRs and side effects of drugs are considered an iatrogenic disease. *Iatrogenic* is a term used when a physician harms a patient as a direct result of treatments—from misdiagnosis of the ailment or from adverse drug reactions used to treat the illness (drug reactions are the most common cause).

How and Why It Happens

ADRs happen when doctors do not spend enough time with their patients to understand their histories, fail to heed warning signs, fail to ask the patient about known allergies to drugs, are not trained well enough to know the ADRs of the drugs they prescribe, or are overworked and fatigued.

Many other aspects contribute to adverse drug reactions, including

- high doses of drugs prescribed without considering the patient's weight and kidney function;
- questionable combinations of drugs that should not be prescribed in conjunction with other drugs;
- the use of high-risk drugs that commonly cause drug-related illness including cardiovascular drugs, cancer drugs, psychotropic drugs (tranquilizers and antidepressants), and anti-inflammatory drugs; and
- excessive treatment duration or drug interactions with food.

Unnecessary use and overuse of antibiotics accounts for millions of pounds of antibiotics used in the United States every year. This amount is enough to give every person ten teaspoons of pure antibiotics per year. It is well documented that exposure to this steady stream of antibiotics has altered the pathogens *Streptococcus pneumonia* and *Staphylococcus aureus* to name a few. Almost all upper respiratory infections are viral and should not be treated with antibiotics. Nevertheless, millions of antibiotics are prescribed annually for viral infections, and many patients with upper respiratory tract infections in the United States still receive antibiotics from their doctor.

Drug-induced cognitive impairment or delirium is caused by commonly used medications that can induce psychiatric symptoms in non-psychiatrically ill patients, especially the elderly. The drugs most often associated with the development of drug-induced dementia are benzodiazepines and anticholinergics. Psychotropic drugs funnel billions of dollars into the psychiatric industry, and many people die every year because of adverse effects to these drugs. Some doctors and rehabilitation staff believe it is easier to manage a sedated patient rather than understand and deal with the patient in his or her true mental state. This happened two times during Mom's hospital and rehabilitation stay.

After eleven weeks in the cardiac intensive care unit, Mom relocated to a local rehabilitation center. She was unable to eat, walk, or transfer by herself, so daily physical and occupational therapy was prescribed. She was scared and uncertain about her footing and progressed slowly. The therapist had no patience for a recovery at her pace. To accelerate her progress, he recommended anti-anxiety medication. The doctors agreed and convinced me to believe this action was needed. So began the parade of experiments. One drug followed another until Mom was so confused that she saw bugs crawling on the wall, people climbing through the window in the middle of the night, singing nurses, and on and on. It reached the point where it backfired and actually stood in the way of her therapy progress. In the meantime, her heart health became compromised, and she was rushed back to the cardiac intensive care.

Upon Mom's return to the hospital, the nurses who treated her previously, noticed the difference in her state of mind. Instead of questioning the psychotropic drugs as the reason, they took it upon themselves to call for a psychiatric evaluation. One afternoon, three well-dressed men descended upon Mom's room to observe and ask questions. They asked me to leave, but I stood outside within earshot. When finished, they discussed their findings with me. The oldest doctor said, "When we asked your mom if she ever thought about dying, she said yes." He raised his eyebrows as if that was a shocking and revealing answer.

I answered with tears in my eyes, "We've been here for nearly four months just barely hanging on. Ask me if I think about dying, and I will tell you yes too." With that, he advised the addition of yet another antidepressant drug to her already large concoction of medications. He scribbled on his notepad and the three walked off, leaving me crying in the hallway.

I immediately went to the nurse in charge and firmly insisted that no new antidepressant be added to Mom's current drug regime until I had a conversation with the one cardiologist I trusted. The next morning I expressed my concerns about the present anti-anxiety medications and the proposed antidepressants. I suggested to slowly wean her off the anxiety drugs to see if that would bring her back to her former lucid state of mind. Fortunately he agreed, and in a few weeks the bugs were gone, the nurses stopped singing and Mom was back to her normal mental status.

These situations occurred because it was more convenient for the therapy staff to work with a drugged patient and because of the narrow focus of the psychiatric specialists. No one paid attention to her needs, which were in fact normal given the situation. Because of the reactions to the anxiety drugs, Mom's therapy progress was delayed by weeks, and her bedsore grew in size because she was confined in bed again.

Finally, it is important to know that there is no way to confirm the actual numbers of adverse drug reactions or side effects of drugs. Doctors are not required by any law to report their knowledge of such cases. This lack of sharing information only perpetuates the problem.

What to Look For

- A quick or rushed doctor who immediately prescribes a drug without discussing the reasoning for the drug or the potential side effects, without inquiring about any known allergies or does not question your use of multiple drugs that might interact negatively with each other

- The use of anticholinergics, antihistamines, antibiotics, psycho-tropics, and many over-the-counter medications that can cause unwanted psychiatric effects or the use of other high-risk drugs (e.g., cardiovascular drugs, cancer drugs and anti-inflammatory drugs) that commonly cause drug-related illness
- Older persons who are frail, cognitively impaired, on multiple drugs, and have kidney or liver insufficiency
- Young children, infants and frail elderly whose low body weight cannot support a normal adult dose
- Signs and signals including a rash; change in respiratory rate, heart rate, hearing, or mental state; seizures; difficulty breathing; diarrhea; or fever

How to Protect Yourself

Tell each doctor or staff person about any known allergic reactions you have had to drugs in the past. Ask about any potential conflicts between the new drug and others that you currently take. Ask your doctor why he or she chose a particular drug, how to take the drug, what danger signs to look for, and if other options exist. Ask not only how effective the drug is but also how well it is tolerated.

Read the insert that accompanies the drug. Know the side effects ahead of time. Share that information with your advocate, a close friend, or a family member. Then, if you happen to experience an adverse effect, someone else can quickly identify the source.

Certain drugs lose their effectiveness if taken with certain foods; other drugs can cause high blood pressure when taken with particular foods. Grapefruit and other seemingly healthy foods can cause some medications to become toxic, making it important to verify that snacks from visitors or home are compatible with the drugs you take.

If you are prescribed an antibiotic, ask if that is the only choice or the least offensive choice in relation to potential side effects. Don't accept a quick yes answer. Dig deeper, ask questions, and be informed. And do not fall into the advertising trap of believing you have a problem just because you saw it on television. Think twice before you go to your doctor to request a drug you may not need.

As much as there is bad information on the Internet, there is also a lot of accurate self-policing that goes on through forums, blogs, and other consumer-driven websites. Check reputable sources on the Internet before you take any prescribed or over-the-counter medicines to look for potential or known problems with the drug. Many informative websites offer comprehensive lists of drugs, pictures, and an interaction checker.

The website, *Drugs.com* lists each drug and states if the interaction risk is high, moderate, or minor. When I type in the drug BuSpar, one of the anti-anxiety medications prescribed for my mom, it shows 691 drug interactions. When I click on each of those 691 drugs, it explains if the interaction is high, meaning the risk of interaction outweighs the benefit; moderate, which says to use it only under special circumstances; or minor, which suggests to assess the risk and consider an alternative drug.

When I visit the list of 691 drugs that react negatively with BuSpar and select Cymbalta, for example, it shows me that taking these two drugs at the same time is a high risk. The page also informs me not to consume alcohol or grapefruit juice when taking this drug. Is your doctor this thorough with you?

Misdiagnosis, Medical Test Mistakes and Harmful Diagnostic Tools

A diagnosis is an educated guess. Doctors derive this guess by reviewing the set of symptoms and any test results. Although tests are an important diagnostic tool, they are not without hazard. Not only can a test be performed incorrectly; the result can be interpreted incorrectly too. Many times the test results are inconclusive, so interpretation and supposition come into play.

As it all becomes more vague—drugs, procedures, and surgeries are thrown into the mix in an attempt to determine the problem. Each test, treatment, and intervention comes with its own potential for error. The more tests you have, the greater margin there is for a mistake; meanwhile, you may not get the treatment for the condition you do have, or subjected to risky treatments for problems you do not have.

Some tests can be hazardous. X-rays have serious consequences because of exposure to radiation. Even though the dose is small, the effect is cumulative, and the damage adds up, increasing your risk of cancer. This is not to say that X-rays and CT scans aren't sometimes needed. If you think the test might be unnecessary or potentially hazardous, be sure to discuss your concerns with your doctor.

The Joint Commission issued a publication titled *Radiation risks of diagnostic imaging*. In the report, they say,

> Diagnostic radiation is an effective tool that can save lives. The higher the dose of radiation delivered at any one time, however, the greater the risk for long-term damage. If a patient receives repeated doses, harm can also occur as the cumulative effect of those multiple doses over time. Conversely, using insufficient radiation may increase the risk of misdiagnosis, delayed treatment, or if the initial test is inadequate, repeat testing with the attendant exposure to even more radiation. The risks associated with the use of ionizing radiation in diagnostic imaging include cancer, burns and other injuries. X-rays are officially classified as a carcinogen by the World Health Organization's International Agency for Research on Cancer, the Agency for Toxic Substances and Disease Registry of the Centers for Disease Control and Prevention, and the National Institute of Environmental Health Sciences. Over the past two decades, the U.S. population's total exposure to ionizing radiation has nearly doubled. Diagnostic imaging can occur in hospitals, imaging centers, physician and dental offices and any physician can order tests involving exposure to radiation at any frequency, with no knowledge of when the patient was last irradiated or how much radiation the patient received. (2011)

A deadly form of misdiagnosis involves heart health. Heart attacks have a high misdiagnosis rate, especially for women. Numerous findings show that doctors are more likely to miss critical heart problem warning signs in female patients than in male patients. Specifically, older women have a greater chance for misdiagnosis and are frequently sent home from the hospital. Once home, their chances of dying from heart complications double.

Mom was in recovery from her reverse total shoulder replacement when she had a heart attack. The ECG at 10:53 AM showed a problem. At 4:30 PM cardiology recognized she was in fact having a severe myocardial infarction. For at least five and a half hours, and most likely longer, Mom endured a heart attack. As they say with any kind of heart situation, time is muscle and her heart muscle was severely compromised. Because of this missed diagnosis, she underwent several salvage surgeries including stents, a coronary artery bypass graft, and the insertion of a right ventricular assist device—a small pump that substitutes for the normal heart. The question is how could a trained staff of anesthesiologists, nurses, and assistants all miss the obvious clues? Even a third-grade child could read the ECG report that stated in words, "heart attack in progress." The lesson here is that misdiagnosis and missed diagnosis happens.

Misdiagnosis rates in the ICU have been studied, with rates ranging up to 40 percent. The prevalence of misdiagnosis is widespread, yet many people never realize they have been victims. Reports show that nearly one in six people have been misdiagnosed at some point in their medical history. Scary stuff!

Another way to think about hospital misdiagnoses is to remember the law of the instrument. When you talk to a surgeon, the problem and solution will most likely involve surgery. Talk to a holistic practitioner and he or she might point to therapies, herbs, and lifestyle changes. So, it is imperative to get several opinions from reputable sources before deciding upon a form of action that might only speak to the preference or inclination of the person making the recommendation.

What It Is

A misdiagnosis is a wrong diagnosis. Considered a medical error, a misdiagnosis can occur by diagnosing the patient with the wrong condition, failing to diagnose anything at all or delaying diagnosis and allowing complications to develop.

How It Happens

Doctors make mistakes in diagnoses, including:

- failure to take a patient's complaints seriously or to notice or understand the nature of a patient's symptoms;
- failure to refer a patient to a specialist for further testing or treatment;
- ordering the wrong test, misunderstanding the test results, or misreading lab reports;
- poor X-rays and other imaging errors;
- relying exclusively on technology or the use of test results exclusively to make a diagnosis;
- getting the results too late to give you the best treatment;
- improper labeling of specimens; and
- lack of focus, fatigue, and rushed and harried behavior on the part of the doctor

What to Look For

- Test results that don't match with the diagnosis
- Treatment that does not work as expected
- A doctor who is brief, rude, defensive, vague or doesn't pay attention to what you have to say
- Radical, immediate surgery or treatment suggestion
- A gut feeling on your part that something is not right

How to Protect Yourself

To ensure solid test results, ask your doctor these series of questions:

- What should you know about my health?
- Should I avoid certain foods or drinks before or after the test and for how long?
- Should I take my usual medicine before the test?
- Is there anything else I need to do to prepare for the test?
- Is the test accurate? What is the error rate?
- What are the chances for false-positive or false-negative errors?

After the test, get a copy of the results and read them using the Internet as a guide to explain words you don't understand. Learn how to decipher your blood test results. Keep all copies to compare to see if changes occur for the better or the worse.

Additional questions to ask your doctor about your diagnosis and potential tests and exams include, how sure are you of the diagnosis? What else could it be? Is there anyone else with whom we should consult?

If the treatment does not work, reconsider the diagnosis and get a second opinion. Always look for a second or even a third opinion if the first diagnosis or treatment options seem drastic. If the doctor is short with his or her time or if he or she is vague, demand answers until you are satisfied—or change doctors.

Patients most prone to harm from diagnostic radiation are children, young adults, pregnant women, those with diabetes mellitus and hyperthyroidism, and individuals receiving multiple doses of radiation. The diagnostic procedures associated with radiation doses are CT scans and nuclear medicine namely a PET scan, which uses radioactive substances for picture taking and fluoroscopy—a technique for obtaining "live" X-ray images.

It is especially important to question all radiology reports. To reduce your exposure to ionizing radiation, ask if ultrasound, MRI or other imaging techniques can be used with equal results. If not, ask for the lowest dose possible and wear protective radiation shields. Ask about the machine's maintenance history and if your technician is trained and has experience with that particular model.

Ask if the images and biopsies are clear enough to read and interpret with accuracy. Did your doctor speak directly to the radiologist or technician who read and interpreted the report, or is the doctor merely reading a copy of the report? Did the images rule out the problem, or did the images simply fail to show the problem? If the latter is the case, perhaps the problem didn't show up on the image because of poor positioning or technologist error.

If something is wrong or inconclusive, have another radiologist or technician interpret the results—from a group independent from the first, to ensure a nonbiased reading. Keep track of all radiation exams.

Try to avoid repeated exams due to poor image quality or unavailable reports from prior exams.

Be proactive when it comes to finding out your test results. Don't assume that no news is good news. You have every right to request and receive information about your test results.

Ask these questions before you leave the testing site: When will the results be ready? How will my doctor and I be informed of the results? Can you give me a telephone number to call if I have questions? If you are told that you will not hear anything unless there is a problem, ask for a phone call, no matter what the results say. Get a day and time to expect the call and the name and number of the person to contact should the time pass and you do not get the phone call. If no one calls at the designated time, call them and keep calling until you get the results. Once you receive the verbal results, ask for a printed copy for your file.

To be certain the test you get is the one ordered by your doctor, get a copy of the order from your doctor, and take it to the test. If you think you are about to get the wrong test, don't be afraid to tell the staff. During any lab exams, ask to see the labels on the containers of your lab samples. The labels should have your full name and date of birth. Make sure the containers are immediately sealed to prevent mislabeling and contamination.

After every test, follow up with the doctor who ordered the test to review the results. For all of you shy and gentle folks, remember this is not being a pain in the butt or trying to push or hurry someone. This is you managing your health and your life. What else could be more important?

Unnecessary Tests and Procedures

Because doctors are concerned about being sued, they may practice defensive medicine, meaning they might order unnecessary tests to prove they have done their due diligence and have explored every avenue. Aside from the financial cost either to your or the insurance company, many invasive tests come with some sort of risk. As an educated health consumer or patient advocate, it is necessary to question all recommended tests.

What It Is

Tests are important tools used to diagnose, confirm, or track your condition. However, doctors may order tests as "routine" or because standards deem them appropriate. Other times tests are ordered to avoid any potential malpractice suits. Frequently, during a hospital stay, the same tests are ordered every day.

How and Why It Happens

Good insurance may result in over testing. If Medicare, Workers' Compensation, or a strong insurance plan is footing the bill, some doctors and hospitals bill all they can to maximize profits. For example, when our neighbor, Ben, turned sixty-five, he scheduled his "free" introduction to Medicare exam with his primary care physician. This exam is available to all Medicare recipients once they reach age sixty-five. A month later, the bill arrived with an added amount of $350. Ben called the doctor to question the fee. The doctor told him, "As I remember, during the exam I asked if you were experiencing any problems, and you said your ankle swells up occasionally whenever you fly."

Ben said, "Yes, I told you that because you asked, but that is not why I came to see you. In fact, I made it clear to your secretary that I was only coming because of the free Medicare exam." "Oh," the doctor snapped, "because we did discuss your ankle, I added that to get more out of Medicare." This is a true and despicable story! It is also called "upcoding," when a provider exaggerates the level of service performed.

In addition to upcoding—doctors, labs and hospitals may also unbundle a service or a test to create additional revenue. "Unbundling" happens when a provider breaks one medical event into individual parts. For example, a complete blood count uses a single blood draw to test for many components and should be billed as one event. Unbundling separates each test and bills for each one. Upcoding and unbundling are two fraudulent acts used to increase provider revenue, making an unnecessary test even more lucrative.

Medical tests also account for the largest portion of a hospital bill and are the most expensive. Medical tests provide the greatest source of income for hospitals, which is why many of them demand that every patient undergo a series of tests upon admission, even though the tests may have been performed the day before in a doctor's office or laboratory.

Sometimes just because the technology is available, tests are ordered to use the equipment. When physicians and medical centers buy expensive X-ray, MRI, and CAT scan equipment, they must perform many tests to pay for that equipment. The Office of Technology Assessment was an office of the United States Congress active from 1972 to 1995; its purpose was to provide Congress with in-depth technical assessments to support congressional decision making. They concluded that hospitals, physician-entrepreneurs and medical device manufacturers have approached MRI and CT as commodities with high-profit potential. Many times the decision to purchase and use these devices are influenced by financial outcomes and not appropriate patient selection.

A friend of mine, who owns many medical buildings, corroborates this conclusion. One of his prospective renters asked him to invest in the MRI, a highly technical and expensive piece of medical equipment. When my friend attempted to discuss and discover how long it would take to recoup his investment, the prospective renter told him, "We will scan cats, dogs, and anyone who walks in the door, if they need it or not." My friend politely declined.

Defensive medicine is also all about business. Studies of private sector physicians show that nearly all physicians admit to practicing defensive medicine. Doctors walk a fine line and must be concerned about defending their actions and decisions. When patients demand testing that their friends have had or that they've heard about on television or the Internet, without fully understanding the purpose or ramifications of the test—doctors may attempt to protect themselves by agreeing to the test.

What to Look For

- Daily testing of the same test or a vague answer to why the test is needed. If you ask a nurse or other care provider why you are having the test and they say, "Because the doctor ordered it," ask to speak with the ordering doctor personally. You have every right to know about a test before testing and to understand why the test is being performed.

- Doctors who do not make the time to listen to what you have to say. The process of diagnostic elimination is much easier and more profitable, so they simply order a battery of tests. This places the burden and risks on patients and the insurance companies.
- A specialist or another treating doctor who does not know your history or has not seen your test results, a new treating doctor who wants to order his or her own set of redundant tests, or a younger physician who is likely to prescribe medical tests as a substitute for experience.

How to Protect Yourself

Choose your doctor with care. Be sure to understand his or her philosophy about the use of medical tests. Look for open communication and a willingness to value your input.

Medical tests results are similar to pieces of a puzzle. If you leave out important pieces, there will never be enough of the correct pieces to complete the puzzle. It is your responsibility to be straightforward right from the beginning. Be specific about your symptoms, diet, lifestyle, and exercise habits. Now is not the time to lie about any drug or alcohol use or any other risky behaviors.

When a medical test is ordered, ask the following questions. Your doctor should clarify the reason and explain what he or she is looking for. If your doctor can't give you this information, get a second opinion.

- What else could this illness be?
- Why do I need this test?
- How is the test done?
- What information will the test provide? What will the test rule out? What won't it rule out?
- Will the test be repeated to confirm the diagnosis?
- Is this test the only way to find out that information?
- What are the benefits and risks of having this test?

- How long will it take to get the results, and how will I get them?
- What is the next step after the test?

Keep a file folder of written test results and bring copies with you to doctor appointments and hospital stays to avoid duplication due to unavailability of previous results. I know the consequences of not following this piece of advice firsthand. Before Mom's shoulder surgery, she had several tests, including an ECG, to serve as clearance for surgery. After the shoulder surgery, while having a dramatic heart attack in recovery, I watched the nursing staff scramble for a copy of this ECG to use as a baseline to compare with the current ones. No one sent the ECG results to the surgery center before the operation. I watched as one nurse attempted to reach Mom's primary care physician by phone to see if he had a copy. Sadly, it was late in the afternoon, and the doctor had gone home for the day. It would have been helpful if I had a file folder with me with all of her current test results.

If you are concerned with any radiology or biopsy reports, get copies of your films and take them to an independent radiologist. Images may be unclear and biopsy samples insufficient. Do not hesitate or feel embarrassed to get another informed judgment call, especially if the first opinion will subject you to surgery or other drastic and invasive procedures.

Miscommunication

Enter any hospital and you see the same thing: doctors, nurses, and orderlies running in and out of rooms, back and forth through hallways, and up and down elevators with hundreds of things on their minds. Papers, files, and charts abound. Visitors and guests roam the floors. It is a stressful and chaotic environment, and it is apparent that a level of disorganization exists. Add long hours, exhaustion, and constant unexpected situations, interruptions, and distractions and you have ingredients for tragic results for both patients and hospital staff.

It is easy to see how miscommunication happens. In fact, miscommunication remains a significant cause of medical malpractice today. With thousands of patients entering and exiting the hospital on a daily basis, it becomes easy for hospitals to sometimes mix up charts or read the chart or prescription incorrectly. If a patient has multiple doctors, there could also be miscommunication as to who is handling which treatment. That means you could be treated twice or not treated at all.

The Joint Commission issued a report titled *What Did the Doctor Say?—Improving Health Literacy to Protect Patient Safety* that addresses another noteworthy area of concern:

Health literacy issues and ineffective communications place patients at greater risk of preventable adverse events. If a patient does not understand the implications of her or his diagnosis and the importance of prevention and treatment plans, or cannot access healthcare services because of communications problems, an untoward event may occur. The same is true if the treating physician does not understand the patient or the cultural context within which the patient receives critical information. Cultural, language and communication barriers—together or alone—have great potential to lead to mutual misunderstandings between patients and their healthcare providers.

When literacy collides with health care, the issue of "health literacy" begins to cast a long patient safety shadow. Health literacy is defined as the degree to which individuals have the capacity to obtain, process, and understand basic health information and services needed to make appropriate health decisions. Most Americans (44 percent) fall into the "intermediate" level of prose literacy. That is, they can apply information from moderately dense text and make simple inferences. Yet, health care information – such as insurance forms, consent forms and medication instructions – is often very complex and seemingly impenetrable. Even those who are most proficient at using text and numbers may be compromised in the understanding of health care information when they are challenged by sickness and feelings of vulnerability.

According to the Institute of Medicine, there is more to health literacy than reading and understanding health information. Health literacy also encompasses the educational, social and cultural factors that influence the expectations and preferences of the individual, and the extent to which those providing health care services can meet those expectations and preferences. Health care practitioners literally have to understand where their patients "are coming from" – the beliefs, values, and cultural mores and traditions that influence how health care information is shared and received. Addressing health literacy issues is not the sole burden of those providing services. There are implications as well for health care policymakers, purchasers and payers, regulatory bodies, and health care consumers themselves. (2007)

What It Is

At the end of every shift, the outgoing nurses sit down with the incoming ones for ten to fifteen minutes to discuss their patients' care. This is their opportunity to share the important events of the shift, patients' conditions and symptoms, important laboratory results, and anything else that might affect the patients' care for the next shift. This is called a change of shift report better known as the "handoff."

There is a scary collapse in communication during patient handoffs. The majority of serious medical errors involve miscommunication between hospital staff when patient responsibility is transferred. Breakdowns happen between doctors or between nurses at the end of a shift and at the start of a new one; between doctors and nurses; between a primary care physician and specialist; and between locations. Any time you have a change in staff or scenery, be aware of the potential for handoff miscommunication. In addition to patient harm, defective handoffs can lead to delays in treatment, unsuitable treatment, and increased time in the hospital.

Health care organizations have long struggled with the process of passing necessary and critical information about a patient from one caregiver to the next, or from one team of caregivers to another. Barriers to effective handoffs include incomplete information, too many delays, not returning calls, inability to take the report because of workload or competing priorities, lack of opportunity to discuss the handoff, and lack of a handoff at all. At the Joint Commission's Center for Transforming Healthcare Press Conference for Hand-off Communications, Mark Chassin, President states:

> This communication between caregivers when responsibilities for patient care is transferred or handed off plays a role in an estimated 80 percent of serious preventable adverse events. It is an ubiquitous problem. Each time a patient moves from one area of care to another; for example, from the emergency department to a medical surgical in-patient unit, from an ICU to an in-patient unit, from a recovery room to an in-patient unit, or from one set of providers to another during a change in shift; those are transitions of care which we informally refer to as hand-offs. Hand-offs are critical because important information about patients' histories, the exact condition they have, their stability or instability, their treatment; all of that information is needed to appropriately care for the patients and that information can get lost or garbled in transition. One study estimated that in a typical teaching hospital there are 4,000 patient hand-offs every day or 1.6 million per year. When you think about those staggering numbers, you get an idea of how many opportunities there are for miscommunication. (2010)

How It Happens

Miscommunication can happen when a doctor gets interrupted or distracted when ordering or writing a prescription, treatment, or diagnosis; when the staff is overworked and tired; when handoffs are incomplete or non-existent; when there is a high patient-to-nurse ratio; or because of something as simple as sloppy handwriting. Too many people involved with care can cause a lack of continuity.

An example of miscommunication between a doctor's orders and the dietary staff occurred with regularity during Mom's hospital stay. She was diagnosed with a swallowing disorder called dysphagia. She was also a high risk for aspiration pneumonia—when food or liquids are breathed into the lungs or airways leading to the lungs. Because of this, the use of a drinking straw was prohibited, as it would have encouraged a quick and direct deposit to places where liquid should not gather.

Morning after morning a straw arrived with her breakfast tray despite the menu card that accompanied the meal that said NO STRAW. This could have been a deadly mistake had I not been present. Weeks later at the rehabilitation center, the straw situation continued. Every morning I found a glass of water with an open straw brought in by the night nurse. Despite taping a sign to the bed tray, I could not solve the straw problem.

Miscommunication can also be caused by hierarchy attitudes. High-level doctors and surgeons or arrogant nurses can sometimes intimidate their underlings by appearing bothered or behaving rudely or responding with anger when approached for clarifications and questions. This can result in reduced communication and a lack of information transfer in an effort "not to bother so and so." Lack of respect between sender and receiver; differences of protocol between microsystems—departments, floors, and facilities; or cultural differences, whether it be language, customs, or focus can also cause miscommunications.

Too many anesthesiologists involved in the administration of anesthesia can also cause issues. A presurgical exam of the patient may involve a nurse anesthetist and anesthesiologist, yet the surgical anesthesiologist may be someone different. The anesthesiologist in charge is responsible for a written anesthesiology plan before any anesthetic medication is administered, and all relevant parties are to read and understand the plan. However, absence of a written plan or deviation of written protocols do happen, making it easy for others involved with the administration of anesthesia to make an error.

Another area of hospital miscommunication that can cause problems is in the scheduling of surgery. Sometimes patients are prepared for surgery when a surgeon is not available or there is a lack of support staff for the operating team because of a scheduling miscommunication.

Another cause of miscommunication can occur if you are picked up and transported by emergency medical services (EMS). The EMS may hastily give an inaccurate report to the hospital about symptoms and the treatment performed en route. This could result in a double dose or no dose of an appropriate treatment.

In addition to miscommunication between health care professionals, miscommunication can also happen between patients and health care professionals. For example, patients with limited literacy may find it difficult to navigate the health care system. They may feel intimidated to ask for help or are embarrassed to admit they do not read well or understand. People with low health literacy tend to be hospitalized more frequently and for longer periods. Because doctors squeeze more patients into their workday, patients with limited literacy skills who need more time are at risk for not getting the attention and time they need because of this communication difficulty.

What to Look For

- Too many doctors and staff in your room at the same time
- A change of staff or a shift change
- A change of scenery—moving from ICU to another floor, from emergency to a hospital care unit, from your room to a testing area or treatment room (A change of scenery usually involves a change of staff making the opportunity for miscommunication twice as possible.)
- Tired, exhausted, and yawning staff or those who work a double shift
- An over-talkative staff member who is more interested in jabbering rather than paying attention to your details
- A staff member who is interrupted by another staff member
- A brief, rushed, rude, or harried staff member who does not take the time to "hear" you or who speaks in a language or with an accent you cannot consistently understand
- A staff member who uses too much jargon or medical terms, is ambiguous on purpose, or is insensitive to your culture or health literacy

How to Protect Yourself

Determine early on who is responsible and in charge of your care and clear all new proposals with this person. To avoid handoff miscommunication, ask your nurse to tell the next nurse about a problem or request you might have or tell the incoming nurses yourself about any concerns or symptoms you have. If your room has a message board, write notes to your doctor or nurse so they see it upon entering the room. You might be asleep or forget important thoughts when they come in, so write them down in a prominent place. If your room does not have a message board, ask your advocate to bring one in for you. In the meantime, keep a list by your bed. This way you can ask all of your questions at one time.

If you are having surgery, ask to meet your lead anesthesiologist. This person should be with you before, during, and after surgery to ensure continuity of care. If you cannot understand the language or accent of the person speaking to you or if you need an interpreter, ask for one before you consent for testing, medications, or procedures.

Finally, bring this book and the safety logs with you to the hospital for reference. Your attention to the details can help mitigate potential miscommunication mishaps.

Surgery and Complications

Mistakes can happen during surgery. Surgeons can do the wrong surgery; they can operate on the wrong part of your body; or they can operate on the wrong person or perform the wrong surgical procedure. Do not assume your surgical team knows what procedure they are doing and on what part of your body. Be especially mindful if you are having surgery on one of a pair of body parts—arms, feet, knees, kidneys, lungs, breast, or eyes.

And just like the dramatic hospital television shows, surgical teams can forget to remove clamps and sponges before closing the surgical site, although there is not much you can do about this.

What It Is

The Joint Commission has a manual titled *Sentinel Event Policy and Procedures* that outlines many unexpected, adverse events involving death; serious physical or psychological injury; or the risk thereof. These events are called *sentinel* because they signal the need for immediate investigation and response. Those events on the list that fall under the heading of surgery and complications are

- blood transfusion reaction involving administration of blood or blood products having major blood group incompatibilities;
- surgical and nonsurgical invasive procedures performed on the wrong patient or wrong site;
- the wrong procedure performed on a patient; and
- unintended retention of a foreign object in a patient after surgery or other procedure.

According to The Joint Commission's *Sentinel Event Data reports*, the most prevalent sentinel events over the past few years have been unintended retention of a foreign object in a patient after surgery or other procedure; delay in treatment; and wrong patient, wrong site, or wrong procedure. The Joint Commission also studies the root causes of these sentinel events and shows that poor leadership and poor communication are the top causes for nearly every undesirable outcome (2011). So this is not me making up frightening material just to shock you. If The Joint Commission has a policy and procedure manual for sentinel events, these things happen with enough frequency to warrant intervention.

How and Why It Happens

Mistakes can happen for a variety of reasons. Here are a few situations that lend themselves to a potential mistake, many of which point to poor leadership and lack of communication:

- human error caused by haste, carelessness, ignorance, exhaustion, or poor judgment calls—wrong X-rays picked up before surgery or inserted backward into the lighted view box or a nursing aide who preps or drapes the wrong side of the patient
- insufficient anesthesia
- an overworked, overtired team performs an emergency surgery at a late hour

- multiple surgeons operate and/or multiple procedures are performed at the same time
- a last-minute surgeon or staff change or emergency surgery where the surgeon is not well prepared
- a surgeon performing a procedure that he or she has not expertly mastered or a fairly new procedure or technology
- overuse of technology, leading to still more treatment

What to Look For

Before your surgery, look at your surgical team. If they appear rushed, tired, haggard, or groggy, tell them your concern.

As irritating as it is for multiple people to ask your name repeatedly, it truly is a good thing. Recently, Mom went back to the hospital for an overnight surgery. The morning of the surgery, in the pre-surgery holding area, a young man walked over to her bed with a bag of IV fluid. As he prepared to hang it on her IV pole, Mom asked, "What is that for?" He replied, "It's just something for your back surgery." Mom sat up in shock and replied, "I'm not having back surgery." With arrogance, the young man answered, "Yes you are, it's written on the board."

This is why everyone associated with your care is supposed to verify the information on your identification bracelet so that you are who they think you are. Likewise, someone should review the pre-surgery informed consent form with you to confirm the kind of surgery you will have, explain the risks of your surgery, answer any questions you may have, and that you agree to have the surgery.

How to Protect Yourself

Before you enter the operating room, you or your advocate should see the surgeon, anesthesiologist, nurses, and staff to go over your name, birth date, type of surgery, and the correct site on your body. Your surgeon should initial the surgery site beforehand. Be sure you are still awake when this happens. If that is not possible, ask your advocate to be there to verify the marking of the site. Ask your surgeon to take a "time-out" just before your surgery to make sure they are doing the right surgery on the right part of your body.

If possible, discuss your anesthesia options days before surgery. Too much anesthesia increases the risk of complications, and yet a staggering number of surgical patients wake up in the middle of their operations because of too little. Ask your surgeon or anesthesiologist to make sure you stay under for the entire operation, and find out if the anesthesiologist will personally administer and monitor you throughout the operation. You have a right to insist that he or she be there at all times during the procedure. This can be included in the informed consent form.

Maintaining a normal body temperature during surgery may help prevent infections. Warming blankets and gowns can control your temperature before, during and after surgery.

If possible, schedule your surgery for well-staffed times—Tuesdays, Wednesdays, or early Thursdays. To get the best postoperative care, avoid surgery times near the weekend or toward the end of the day. Usually the weekend and night staff is sparse.

From personal experience, find out about your heart attack and blood clot risk. A pre-surgical evaluation can tell if you are at risk of having a heart attack or stroke during the operation. If you are, a beta-blocker—metoprolol (Toprol-XL) or atenolol (Tenormin) or other medication may be appropriate before the operation.

After surgery, deep abdominal breathing can ward off pneumonia and other post surgical respiratory complications. You may even get a little breathing "toy" called a handheld "spirometer" to keep your lungs free and clear of fluid buildup that can develop after surgery.

Preventing a surgical mistake happens long before you enter the operating room. You and your advocate have the ability to lessen the chance of an error by implementing many if not all of the suggestions in this chapter.

Pressure Sores

It is much easier to prevent a pressure sore than it is to heal one. Pressure sores can be deadly and are one of the leading causes of death due to hospital treatment and stays. I became an expert on pressure sores during Mom's long hospital visit. She was immobilized for the first month because of the shoulder surgery and subsequent heart problems.

Consequently, she developed a sore on her tailbone area. I was unaware of this until almost the third month into our ordeal. It was then I met the wound care team and had my first look at a hole about the size of Texas!

With all the other challenges Mom faced, I soon realized this had the greatest potential to kill her. For weeks, I watched and learned everything I could about pressure sores. I asked questions each day. At night I researched the Internet for more information. In the end, no assisted living home would accept her because she had a stage four pressure sore. So, upon discharge Mom came to live at my home. On her first day home, a nurse came by with a bag of bandages and other wound-cleaning lotions and potions. I watched as she cleaned and dressed the cavernous wound. Then she said, "I'll be back once a week to check on it." I nervously answered, "Um, doesn't it need to be cleaned and rebandaged every day?" "Oh, yes! You'll be doing that," she said. I was mortified. Being a determined patient advocate, I dealt with the problem directly and over the next few months helped the gaping hole to self-heal. It was an experience as none other, and I must admit I am now well versed on bedsores.

As I learned—acquiring a hospital stay associated pressure sore leads to increased pain for the patient, a longer hospital stay, potential disfigurement, a poorer quality of life, loss of function, increased expenses, and a greater risk of death.

What It Is

A pressure sore, also called a bed sore, appears when a patient is unable to move. The constant pressure on any given spot cuts off circulation, causing the skin and muscle to deteriorate. These lesions, officially known as decubitus ulcers, can involve parts of the body that are not well padded or lie just over a bone. Common sites of pressure sores for people who use a wheelchair are the tailbone or buttocks, shoulder blades, spine, and backs of arms and legs where they rest against the chair. Frequent locations of pressure sores for people confined to a bed are the back or sides of the head, the rim of the ears, shoulders or shoulder blades, hips, the lower back or tailbone, heels, ankles, and the skin behind the knees.

The four stages of pressure sores are defined by the degree of tissue damage observed. The depth of an ulcer is evaluated on a scale from one to four. The higher the number, the deeper the ulcer:

Stage one is the most superficial, indicated by redness that does not subside after the pressure is relieved. The skin may be hotter or cooler than normal, have an odd texture, or be painful. Stage two is damage to the epidermis or outer skin. In this stage, the ulcer looks similar to a blister or abrasion. Stage three involves the full thickness of the skin and may extend into the subcutaneous tissue layer. This layer has a relatively poor blood supply and can be difficult to heal. At this stage, there may be underlying damage that makes the wound much larger than it may seem on the surface. Stage four is the deepest, extending into the muscle, tendon, or even bone.

How It Happens

A very old doctor randomly showed up at Mom's bedside late one afternoon. Apparently he was a bedsore guru of sorts, having written numerous articles on the ins and outs of these nasty wounds. He was delighted to teach me as much as I wanted to learn. He explained that three different tissue forces cause bedsores:

1. *Prolonged pressure*—When skin and the underlying tissues are trapped between bone and a surface; a bed or wheelchair, the pressure may be greater than the pressure of the blood flowing through the vessels that deliver oxygen and other vital nutrients to tissues. Deprived of these critical nutrients—cells of the skin and other tissues are damaged and may die.

2. *Friction*—Fragile skin is vulnerable to injury. When a person changes position or is handled by care providers, the skin may be dragged across the bed sheets or other surface. Friction causes the surface of the skin to rub away faster than it can be replaced, especially if the skin is moist. For example, when a patient calls for a bedpan and in haste, the nursing staff drags already compromised tailbone skin across sheets, or stuffs and pushes a bedpan across weak and fragile skin, damage can occur.

3. *Shear*—Shear, or the pulling of skin in opposite directions,

happens when a hospital bed is elevated at the head. As the patient slides down in bed, the tailbone moves down, yet the skin over the bone may stay in place. Skin pulled sideways over muscle or bone when moving can stretch and block the blood vessels, restricting blood flow to skin. This motion may damage tissue and blood vessels, making the area more vulnerable to damage from constant pressure. Excessive shearing can affect deeper tissues. Tissue death, or necrosis, begins on the inside and moves outward.

What to Look For

A person with limited mobility or is unable to change positions when seated or in bed is at risk of developing pressure sores. Immobility can be caused by sedation, recovery after surgery, paralysis, weakness, or coma. The inability to feel pain or discomfort because of these things can cause the patient to be unaware of bedsores or the need to change position. Weight loss and muscle atrophy cause a loss of fat and muscle that can result in less cushioning between bones and the bed or wheelchair.

The skin of older adults is more fragile, drier, thinner, and less elastic than the skin of younger adults, making older folks more vulnerable to damage. Patients suffering from dementia or whose mental acuity is compromised by illness or medication are less likely to heed caution to prevent pressure sores.

Skin that is moist from sweat or urine is more likely to be injured and can increase the friction between the skin and clothing or bedding.

Patients who have muscle spasms or other involuntary muscle movement may have an increased risk of pressure sores from frequent friction or shearing.

Any disease that affects circulation, including diabetes and vascular diseases, may cause pressure areas to receive inadequate blood flow, thereby increasing the risk of tissue damage. Smoking impairs circulation and reduces the amount of oxygen in the blood. As a result, smokers can develop severe wounds, and their wounds heal more slowly.

How to Protect Yourself

Changing positions is the simple key to preventing pressure sores. These position changes need to be frequent, with mindfulness on friction and shear to minimize damage to vulnerable areas.

To Change Positions in a Bed

Reposition every two hours. Use bed linens or a draw sheet to help lift and reposition to reduce friction and shearing. If you have enough body strength, use an assistive device or an overhead trapeze bar to help you change positions. Alternating pressure mattresses and other special rotating beds, foam mattress pads, cushions, or air- or water-filled mattresses can help relieve pressure and protect vulnerable areas from damage. Ask your doctor or nurse about your options. Do not raise the head of the hospital bed more than 30° to prevent shearing. Make sure hospital gowns and sheets are not wrinkled or bunched. Protect bony areas with proper positioning and cushioning. Instead of lying directly on a bone, try to lie at an angle with cushions supporting the back or front. Heels can be cushioned with special inflatable heel protector boots.

To Change Positions in a Wheelchair

Reposition every fifteen minutes. If you have enough body strength, raise your body off the seat by pushing on the arms of the chair, push-up style. If you are unable to move yourself, call an assistant to help at least every hour. Make sure your wheelchair is fitted properly for you and your body type. Special pressure-release wheelchairs tilt to redistribute the pressure and may provide assistance in repositioning and pressure relief. Air- or water-filled, foam, or gel cushions can relieve pressure and help ensure that the body is appropriately positioned in the chair. Ask your physical therapist to help with the selection and placement of wheelchair cushions.

Other strategies to prevent pressure sores include frequent skin inspections, skin care, and good nutrition. It is important to protect and monitor the condition of your skin to identify potential sores and sites.

Ask your nurses to check areas you cannot see or reach. Skin inspection should be a part of routine care for anyone confined to a wheelchair or bed or for anyone with limited ability to reposition. Wash skin with mild soap and warm water and gently dry without rubbing. If assistants bathe you, be sure they use a gentle hand. Keep a bottle of lotion in the room to apply when skin is dry. Manage urinary or bowel incontinence to prevent moisture and bacterial exposure to skin.

Ask your doctor or physical therapist to recommend an appropriate exercise program that improves circulation and builds muscle tissue. To avoid injury, do not attempt any exercises or movements without clearance from your doctor or therapist.

Nutrition, diet, nutritional supplements, and hydration are crucial in the prevention of pressure sores. Check for signs of poor hydration—decreased urine output, darker urine, dry mouth, thirst, dry skin, or constipation. If you need help with eating, be sure that a nurse, assistant, or your advocate is with you during all mealtimes so that you eat sufficient amounts of food.

Evidence shows that a high-protein diet helps healing of sores. A high-protein diet is especially helpful in sores that do not heal in eight weeks. The hospital provided Mom with pure liquid protein during her pressure sore bout, so I bought a bottle to have at home. I needed every tool possible to help heal the cavernous hole. Although I cannot be sure why or how this life-threatening sore came to heal so well, I attribute some of it to the benefits of liquid protein. We used Pro-Stat, produced by Medical Nutrition USA.

An article from their website titled, *Pro-Stat® in the treatment of pressure ulcers* says,

> The Agency for Health Care Policy and Research's (AHCPR) guideline Treatment of Pressure Ulcers notes that studies have linked pressure ulcers and bed sores to malnutrition. Patients need adequate levels of protein, vitamins, and minerals to support wound healing. Inadequate caloric intake can lead to weight loss and use of protein stores for energy instead of healing. According to the AHCPR guideline, patients with pres-

sure ulcers need 30 to 35 kilocalorie and 1.25 to 1.5 grams of protein per kilogram of body weight daily.

Ideally, adequate protein and calories intake may be found through oral intake of food and liquids. For many elderly persons in long-term care the amount of food needed to be consumed for a positive nitrogen balance may be overwhelming, so supplementation is recommended. Supplementation of products that are high in kilocalories and volume may not be able to be tolerated by the aged. Many have decreased appetites and smaller volumes of food must be consumed throughout the day rather than large volumes at one time. Pro-Stat® provides the highest amount of protein in the smallest serving size (15g/30mL) making it easily tolerated by patients with limited appetites. (2011)

It doesn't take long for skin to break down yet pressure sores are slow to heal. The healing process requires meticulous care. Given the hard to reach places where these sores can occur, you may not be able to care for a pressure sore on your own. With improper care, they can become infected and spread infection to the rest of your body. Awareness and early preventive measures are paramount.

Malnutrition

Malnutrition sounds like a problem found in remote or poverty-stricken areas, yet it may be the most unrecognized hospital hazard. It is also easily preventable. However, don't count on the hospital staff to educate you. This is another instance where you need to be proactive.

What It Is

Malnutrition occurs when your body does not get enough nutrients. Signs of malnutrition including fatigue, dizziness, and weight loss can be mistaken for disease, medication side effects, and surgery effects. In the hospital, your nutritional needs are much greater than your needs when you are healthy. Your body needs more protein and calories to help fight infections, heal wounds and incisions, and rebuild strength.

It's a classic complaint that hospital food is bland, tasteless, cold, and usually late in arriving. Compounded with little strength to feed yourself, a weakened appetite, mealtime disruptions, or the inability to reach the food—you have a recipe for a compromised and malnourished body. Malnutrition in hospitals lacks ownership. No one is responsible for this common crisis, so it continues to remain under recognized, under detected, and under managed.

Older patients are at a great risk of not recovering. Fortunately, you or your advocate can help to alleviate this dangerous risk.

How It Happens

Many hospitals have inadequate systems in place to identify patients at risk for malnutrition and either cannot or do not provide appropriate care or consistent monitoring when identified. The initial nutrition screening during admission is hit-and-miss. In a fragmented care system, there is little to no coordination, continuity, or communication between departments and care providers. Nutrition care is not multidisciplinary; the dietitian pops in every now and then, sends a few orders to the kitchen, and that is where it usually ends. Often, not enough trained nutritional support staff are available to assist with mealtimes. Daily weigh-ins are sometimes skipped or sloppily recorded, and in many cases, there are not enough scales per floor. I cannot count how many times I personally ran from hospital floor to floor to retrieve a scale so Mom could monitor her weight each day.

Patients can also have health problems that lead to decreased appetite or trouble eating. A chronic illness, use of certain medications, trouble chewing due to dental issues, problems swallowing, or difficulty absorbing nutrients, and physical or mental limitations can prevent them from eating. To further the problem, hospital menus are not designed for those who have poor appetites or have trouble feeding themselves, and those who eat alone may not enjoy meals, causing skipped meals.

Patients may also have new hospital-implemented dietary restrictions and limits on salt, fat, and sugar. Although such diets are important to manage certain medical conditions, they can also cause food to be tasteless and unappealing. Depression, fear, grief, loneliness, failing health, and lack of mobility may also contribute to a loss of appetite.

What to Look For

- Food left untouched on the meal tray due to an inability to eat without assistance or meals delivered to tables far from a patient's reach
- Signs of poor wound healing, dry skin, easy bruising, dental difficulties, exhaustion, and weight loss, and depression (Nutritional risk is associated with depression in older patients.)
- Medication side effects that directly change appetite, digestion, and nutrient absorption
- Low blood albumin levels and prealbumin levels, which can reflect protein deficiencies and malnutrition

How to Protect Yourself

Before a hospital stay, ask your doctor about starting nutritional supplements, including nutritional drinks and puddings. You can purchase these from drugstores without a prescription. It's smart to be as healthy as you can before entering the hospital. Insist upon nutritional evaluation upon admission and ask for continuous evaluation.

If you must take tests that call for no food or water before the process, make sure your doctor groups all of these tests together so you do not have to fast repeatedly. Inquire about how you will get sufficient nutrients during the fast.

Look for signs and symptoms of malnutrition. Ask for blood test results, and review the following results with your doctor:

For General Screening and Monitoring

- Lipids
- CBC (complete blood count)
- CMP (comprehensive metabolic panel)
- Albumin
- Total protein

For Nutritional Status and Deficiencies

- Prealbumin (decreases in malnutrition, rises and falls rapidly, and can be used to detect short-term response to treatment)
- Iron tests (iron, TIBC and ferritin)
- Vitamin and minerals (B12 and folate, vitamin D, vitamin K, calcium, and magnesium)

Get help with menu selections to assist with meaningful choices. Ask your dietitian about healthy and nutritious snack options to keep in your room. Make sure food trays are within reach.

It is helpful to create a positive atmosphere for your meals. Remove any soiled or dirty linen and close bathroom doors. Play music. Put flowers on your tray. Have your advocate close your door partway to banish hallway clatter. Plan to have someone present for each meal of the day, especially if you need help cutting food, eating, or drinking.

Because of Mom's swallowing disorder, the nutritionist felt it essential to show up for lunch. She used the time to conduct mental quizzes, giving story problems and math riddles while my frail mom attempted to enjoy her meal. It was difficult for her to eat under those circumstances, so lunch consisted of a few bites of cold food. Protect your mealtimes by making the setting conducive to eating: do not allow interruptions, lab work, tests, or evaluations.

Daily exercise, even if it's light, can stimulate appetite and strengthen bones and muscles. Just be sure to get clearance from your doctor before initiating any kind of exercise regime.

Also talk to your doctors about changing medications that affect appetite. Discuss and understand any need for a restricted diet and learn how to make this new diet more interesting and tasty. The food delivered to your room may not follow your dietary needs. It's up to you or your advocate to monitor this.

Dietary modifications and nutritional supplements are by far the easiest and safest way to care for nutritional needs. However, if you need specialized nutrition support, two other routes are applicable. The first is enteral nutrition (EN), a liquid nutrition given through a tube inserted into the nose, down the throat, and into the stomach. This tube is called a nasogastric, or NG, tube. The fluid contains essential nutrients and helps supplement or replace a regular diet. The intestines absorb nutrients from the fluid more easily than from regular food. Feedings may be given during the day or at night during sleep. Enteral nutrition can be delivered through the nasogastric route for temporary feedings. For longer-term feeding, a minor surgical process implants a tube into the pharynx, esophagus, stomach, or intestines.

The second route is total parenteral nutrition (TPN), a liquid nutrition given through a needle that is inserted into a large vein in or near the shoulder, neck, or arm. This method bypasses the digestive tract completely and places nutrients directly into the bloodstream. Complications are possible with both forms and feeding, so you or your advocate should watch for any signs of intolerance or infection.

Finally, you should plan for continuity of nutritional care upon discharge from the hospital.

Equipment Failure and Misuse

The amount of technology used in a hospital is staggering. You are exposed to many medical devices, including IV infusion pumps, heart monitors, X-ray equipment, anesthesia machines, blood pressure machines, and many more. A malfunction in these medical technologies can lead to serious injuries or even death. You have enough to worry about during a hospital stay; machine maintenance and repair should not be on your list. Hopefully the product manufacturers build the machines correctly, and the hospital staff knows how to monitor, maintain, and use them properly.

What It Is

Equipment can fail for many reasons—a product defect, forgotten maintenance, repair problems, dead batteries, operator error, or negligence. Intravenous (IV) pumps; diagnostic cancer equipment; blood pressure equipment; X-ray MRI or CAT scanning machines; and many others may not only fail, they can be used improperly. This may be hard for you to avoid.

How it Happens

Hospital equipment is complex and can fail in many ways. The following are a few common scenarios.

An infusion pump delivers fluids into a patient's body through an IV. Such fluids include medications, nutritional fluids, saline, antibiotics, pain relievers, chemotherapy, insulin, and others. Some of the pumps are positioned bedside, and others are portable. As with anything mechanical, these pumps can experience battery failure, broken parts, software issues, or alarm malfunctions. I remember reading about a particular infusion pump that was recalled because of a defect in design that led to two hundred and seventy reported patient injuries, eight deaths and other non-life-threatening incidents due to drug overdose.

Misuse of technology is also a major issue. Patients have been injured, and others have died because of medical gas mix-ups. This usually happens when the wrong gas is connected to the oxygen supply system. For example, nitrogen gas can be connected to the oxygen gas supply by mistake.

Catheter and tubing misconnections remain a serious problem, so much so that The Joint Commission issued an alert to address tubing misconnections as a persistent and potentially deadly occurrence. A friendly nurse explained to me that there is one standard connector used on many devices that serve completely different functions, thereby increasing the risk of a tubing misconnection. It is easy to see that if many nurses are in the room or if the nurse is tired, distracted, or not well informed, the fluids meant to go into a vein may be inadvertently connected to the stomach tubing or vice versa just because the connector fits.

Although not an equipment failure, the MRI testing room is home to strong magnetic fields that can cause projectile accidents involving equipment in the room. If the oxygen tank in the MRI room is not properly secured, the magnetism of the MRI scanner can attract the metallic tank and lead to a propelled "missile" flying across the room. It sounds remote, yet it's highly possible.

Sometimes in the hustle and bustle of day-to-day demands, staff members may forget to change batteries in pumps and monitors and fail to perform basic machine maintenance. This reminds me of one nurse who religiously turned off the alarms on the IV pumps and bed alarms because she didn't want to hear them.

What to Look For

When you are a patient in the hospital, your job is to get better and get out. You don't want to fret about potential equipment failure. So, your advocate should learn everything about the equipment in your room. He or she doesn't need to be a machine diagnostician, but should at least understand what the machines do, what the alarms sound like, what the alarms mean, and how to read the settings.

If something is wrong, or if a nurse or doctor behaves in an unsure manner while working with the equipment, say something. Document your questions—who you asked and what they said.

How to Protect Yourself

Understand the equipment used in your room. Ask what to expect from the equipment and when and why it makes sounds. Do not touch the dials on the machines or attempt to operate them yourself, and do not let visitors touch the equipment either. Ask your nurse if he or she has used this equipment before and find out if he or she feels comfortable using it.

Do not hesitate to ask your nurse if he or she is sure that the correct tubes are attached correctly. To avoid a medical gas mix-up, remind your nurses to "take a look before you hook" and if it "won't connect, don't connect." In other words, don't try to force something to connect. Be wary if someone tries to connect an adaptor to make a connection work. If in doubt, speak up.

Timing

It is a documented fact that medical mistakes are frequent during certain times of the year and even certain times of day. Similar to the rest of the working world, hospitals have a staff hierarchy, and tenure dictates who gets first dibs on time off for holidays, vacations, and weekends.

What It Is

You cannot predict a health emergency or a hospital visit. However, if you have a choice at all, avoid the summer months. A new study reported in the *Annals of Internal Medicine* by Dr. John Young of the University of California, San Francisco, takes a complete look at death rates and complications occurring in hospitals throughout the year. The study shows that at teaching hospitals responsible for training new doctors, patient death rates increase while competence in patient care decreases during the month of July (2011). In the spring, the most seasoned residents graduate, leaving behind a flock of first year newbies. Medical students become interns, interns become residents, and residents become doctors. By July, these brand new practitioners are just beginning to take care of real patients. To coincide with that, the doctors, nurses, and other support staff with tenure and those with the most experience begin their summer vacations. It comes as no surprise to find that this combination of circumstances not only disrupts patient care, it also escalates medical error rates, increases surgical complications, and causes a plethora of additional undesirable outcomes.

Young's study, which reviewed data from thirty-nine previous studies that tracked health outcomes including death and complications from medical procedures, found that death rates increased up to 34 percent in July. The study also found patients are more likely to experience prolonged stays and more tests in July.

Each year the so-called "July effect" influences about 100,000 staff in teaching hospitals. Young notes that such a dramatic shift in personnel rarely occurs in other industries on such a regular basis. There is also a severe discrepancy in quality between daytime and nighttime inpatient services, and weekday versus weekend care. Many studies confirm that survival rates from in-hospital cardiac arrest are lower during nights and weekends.

How It Happens

If your hospital is a teaching hospital, be aware of the July effect. If your hospital is a nonteaching hospital, you won't have freshman interns filling the hallways. However, the staff with the most tenure and experience usually selects their vacations during the summertime.

Most patients are admitted to the hospital at night or on the weekend. The off hours rarely have senior managers present. Those with the most seniority usually choose to work weekdays. Those with lesser tenure— many of whom have less training and less familiarity with the hospital and its procedures and protocols—work weekends and nights. Because hospitals quiet down at night when patients sleep, hospitals schedule fewer nurses, lowering the nurse-to-patient ratio. Doctors are absent at these times too. All of this adds up to more demands on those who work during these hours. The consequences for patients include higher mortality rates, more surgical complications, more medical errors, and higher readmission rates.

What to Look For

A visit to the hospital during summer months, holidays, weekends, and nights are the most dangerous times for medical errors.

If a procedure is bumped to late in the day, surgeons and staff may be tired and the aftercare crew may be sparse or not as well trained or experienced as the day shift.

How to Protect Yourself

Ask your advocate to be with you as much as possible. If you do not have a family member or a friend to act as an advocate, hire a sitter, companion, or private duty nurse to fill in. Peace of mind is well worth the money.

Try to schedule your surgery early in the morning and early in the week when doctors are fresh, before surgeries become backed up, and when the operating room is at its cleanest. If your surgery is not an emergency, ask to schedule it on a Tuesday, Wednesday, or Thursday morning. This way, your postoperative care will occur midweek when staffing is at full capacity. Lack of staff may cause reduced postoperative care on the weekend.

You have the right to ask your doctors and nurses about their level of training. If you feel uncomfortable with the level of care, speak with

someone you trust before agreeing to any invasive surgery, test, treatment, or medicine change. On several occasions, I asked to have certain
night shift folks removed from my mom's room because of their inability
to handle her delicate and complicated case. Remember, you are not
running for office—not everyone has to like you. The goal is to stay
alive and get out as quickly as possible. You will most likely never see
these people again. If they do not offer quality care, get them out of your
room and off your case.

Falls

I was surprised to learn that falls are the second greatest cause of
accidental deaths after car accidents. Although you feel safe, tucked into
a high-railed hospital bed with call buttons pinned to your gown; most
hospital falls occur in the patient's room or bathroom.

What It Is

You don't have to be old to fall. During a hospital stay, your physical
and mental responses may be diminished. Given a new environment and
an altered state of awareness, it is easy to lose balance and coordination.
Even if a fall doesn't cause a serious injury, it may cause further hospitalization, rehabilitation, or placement in a skilled nursing facility, creating
emotional and financial burdens.

How and Why It Happen

Many falls occur when patients try to get out of bed either to go to
the bathroom or walk around the room by themselves. Here are a few
common reasons why falls happen:

- Patient is weak, tired, ill, or not physically fit, or he or she has
  vision problems.
- Patient is tied to rolling IV poles and delicate catheters.
- Medicines and sedations may cause weakness, sleepiness,
  confusion, or dizziness.
- Threats include slippery or wet floors or stairs, obstructed path-

ways, darkness, a history of prior falls, transfer to a new room, improper footwear, or frequent bathroom visits.

What to Look For

There isn't one environmental reason that contributes to a fall—rather a combination, including the functionality of each individual patient. If you are weak, frail, ill, have compromised vision, or out of balance due to medications, you may be at risk for a fall no matter how safe the physical environment. Your nurse should conduct a risk of falling assessment. Environmental issues—a crowded or cluttered room, bed positioned too high, bed tray, phone, meals, water and other necessities placed out of reach, or staff members who delay in responding to call button requests are hazards your advocate can address and correct.

How to Protect Yourself

If you need to get out of bed, be safe. If you are shaky, use your call button to ask for help. Ask for help when going to the bathroom or walking around the room or in hallways. If you are told to stay in bed, don't get up without help. To safely exit your bed—lower the height of the bed and the side rails, and use the bedrails for support. Sit for a minute on the side of the bed to regain your equilibrium and make sure you are steady. Don't attempt to climb over the rails.

One afternoon, as I walked down the hallway of the hospital, I heard shouting coming from a patient's room. An elderly woman was sandwiched between the mattress and bedrails. The rails were in the up position. Apparently, the gap between the mattress and the bedrails was so large that she landed in between and could not extricate herself from trouble. Be sure to check for this kind of gap. The mattress should be tight against the bed frame and rails.

Make sure your pathway is clear and the floors are not wet. Do not walk barefoot in the hospital. Wear slippers or socks with rubberized feet. Keep your eyeglasses close by. Put frequently used items in easy-to-reach places that do not require stretching or leaning. The Patient Pod listed in the Helping Hands section of this book is a handy tool, perfect for storing these items.

Medications and their side effects can cause imbalance, weakness, and altered thought processes. If your medicine makes you sleepy, dizzy, foggy, or confused, ask your doctor if there is something else you can take or something you can do to reduce these side effects. If you have bladder issues, make the nurses aware of this and ask for a quick response when you call. Use the handrails and grab bars in the bathroom and shower.

Sit in sturdy chairs that have armrests to help when you sit down and stand up. Use care when transferring from bed to chair or wheelchair. If you are using a wheelchair, make sure to lock the wheels before you sit or stand. Recently, Mom fell to the floor in an airport. During the security screening, the transporter told her to stand up without thinking to lock the wheels. The wheelchair flew backward, and Mom fell down.

Many times the orderlies transport you to a location far away from your room and leave you there all alone until it's your turn for the procedure. Have your advocate go with you to all X-rays, scans, and procedures. If you need assistance for any reason, your advocate will be there to help you. Do not attempt to get off the gurney by yourself.

Here is a helpful tip: pin a shrill whistle to your hospital gown or keep a small bell in your bed at all times to use in case of an emergency.

If you are a known risk for falling, ask for a special low bed. During a particularly bizarre episode of drug-induced delirium, Mom attempted to escape from the rehabilitation center during the middle of the night (not that I blame her). A telephone call from a frantic nurse awakened me at home at 3:00 AM. Mom insisted I was trying to get in to her room by way of the window and she had to get out of bed to open it up.

I rushed over to calm her down and asked the night nurse to find the lowest bed on the premises. Then we found extra mattresses to pad the floor all around the bed. The nurses talked about using restraints, but I didn't allow that. I stayed the rest of the night on one of the floor mattresses to monitor the situation.

Most hospitals indicate a risky patient by posting a falling leaf or other picture outside the patient's door to alert the staff. You and your advocate can incorporate fall prevention strategies throughout your hospital stay. What a shame to survive an illness only to suffer the consequences of a preventable fall.

Safety and Security

A hospital is a slice of society. Anyone and everyone can pass through the doors. No one stands guard to check identification. It's difficult to tell the difference between staff members, patients, visitors, volunteers, clergy, repair folks, delivery people, sales reps, or hoodlums looking for vulnerable prey. Hospitals have open-door policies that leave themselves and others subject to many dangerous crimes and hazards, not to mention a multitude of germs and infections.

What It Is

The Joint Commission keeps a Sentinel Event Database that tracks incidents reported by hospitals, including infant abductions, assaults, homicides, and rapes. Numbers do not tell all, as the reporting of most sentinel events to The Joint Commission is voluntary and represents only a small proportion of actual events. Hospital management makes the decision to report incidents, and many incidents go unreported because they don't fall into the hospital's definition of "violence," and others are absent because officials don't want to present the hospital in a negative way. Regardless of reporting issues, it is obvious that a hospital, given its "welcome-all" philosophy, is poised for a criminal event.

The Joint Commission warns that assault, rape, and homicide are consistently among the top ten reported events. High-traffic and high-stress areas—the emergency department and general medical/surgical patient rooms, are susceptible to criminal events. They continue to caution,

> While controlling access to the facility is imperative and ongoing surveillance of the grounds is a necessity, administrators must be alert to the potential for violence to patients by health care staff members. The stressful environment together with failure to recognize and respond to warning signs such as behavioral changes, mental health issues, personal crises, drug or alcohol use, and disciplinary action or termination, can elevate the risk of a staff member becoming violent towards a patient. Though it is a less common scenario, health care workers who deliberately

harm patients by either assaulting them or administering unpre-scribed medications or treatments, present a considerable threat to institutions. (2010)

I was in the hallway of the cardiothoracic intensive care unit and watched a senior physician physically remove an anesthesiologist from a patient's room—ordering him never to enter that room again. I didn't know the reasons, but later learned of the anesthesiologist's ongoing mental health issues and drug use. The state suspended his license. This caused me to realize that staff members can contribute to patient dangers because of their personal issues.

How It Happens

Many times hospitals are located in downtown locations or other large areas where crime rates are already high. Parking lots and garages rank first in hospital crime incidents. These dark and lonely areas make it easy for a thief to hide behind parked cars, either waiting to assault a victim or waiting to steal a car.

With all of the commotion in a hospital and with patients and fami-lies in a vulnerable state, it is an easy place for thieves to achieve success. Twenty-four hour access with no screening procedures encourages a microcosm of society to mix and mingle in an already overcrowded space with lots of nooks and crannies available as hiding places. Mental health patients use the hospital for follow-up visits, which allows poten-tially unstable persons to create unwelcome situations. Intoxicated or drug-addicted patients and visitors may enter undetected by security guards

What to Look For

Emergency departments are most susceptible to violence because of heavy traffic, high stress levels, and the urgent cases they handle. Emergency rooms can harbor patients who are also criminals and may have guns or other weapons in their possession. Intensive care units are also vulnerable because of elevated stress levels among patients and their loved ones.

Beware of dark or desolate areas, parking garages, low activity times, nights and weekends, any suspicious looking characters, or a gut feeling that something isn't right.

How to Protect Yourself

A smiling woman staffed the front desk at Mom's cardiac intensive care unit. On my first day, I stopped at the desk to check in. No one acknowledged me. The woman just smiled. I smiled back and kept walking toward Mom's room. Each day I watched as people wandered in and out, never checking with the desk lady. On several occasions, men in suits and ties approached me, asking about Mom's condition, "Did anything improper occur that might have landed your mother in the ICU?"

Being a cautious person, I declined to answer and watched as they moved on to the next set of beds to chat with the family members of those patients. Later I learned these men were lawyers. I was shocked the hospital allowed this to happen in such a critical care setting. Never mind the audacity of their questions, how many germs did they carry in to the unit?

During one of our family meetings with the staff, I brought up the safety issue, asking why there was a front desk if no one was required to check in. I was sharply answered with, "This is not a prison. We want the community to feel free to come in and out." I was taken aback not so much by the answer as the tone. An entire ward of vulnerable people had nothing to protect them from the weirdness of the outside world. Unconscious patients, devastated and crying family members, and overworked and stressed staff also had to concern themselves with wandering attorneys and who knows what else. This situation stresses the importance of a having a competent patient advocate to act as a 24/7 private duty security guard by each patient's bedside.

To help with these kinds of unwanted visitors, furnish the nursing staff with a list of acceptable visitors and ask them to inform you if someone who is not on the list arrives. Question the presence of anyone who enters your room.

Feel free to report any threats or suspicious events. Use common sense as you would in any public and crowded location. Be extra aware that during a hospital stay—whether you are the patient, advocate, or visitor—you will likely be in an altered state of awareness, so use extra caution.

Going Home

People view discharge as the end of the road. Yes, you made it out alive, however a mismanaged discharge can lead you right back with a readmission. Discharge is a hazardous handoff time when your care transfers to another facility or directly to your home. Charged with emotion and excitement, the family shuffles your belongings out of your room, the car runs in the discharge zone, and nurses hurry to give your final and last-minute instructions. Sketchy and cryptic written instructions are complicated, with no formal procedures and no coordination or continuity protocols. It is time to go, and you are out of there. They say the devil is in the details. If you and your advocate insist on clear, concise, and correct discharge instructions—posthospital problems are largely preventable.

What It Is

An article from the Annals of Internal Medicine, titled, *The Incidence and Severity of Adverse Events Affecting Patients after Discharge from the Hospital* explains:

> Studies prove that 41 percent of discharged patients have a pending test result, with many requiring urgent medical action. To top it off, a survey of the doctors involved showed almost two-thirds of them were unaware of the test results—results that could have changed treatments and management.

> The most common discharge error is medication use. Up to 42 percent of patients do not know how to continue or manage their medications at home. Part of the problem is nearly half of adults have trouble understanding simple health information such as oral instructions or prescription information. Less than half of patients know their diagnoses, treatment plans, or

the side effects of prescribed medications. Discharged Medicare patients return to the hospital within thirty days of discharge close to 20 percent of the time, and two-thirds are readmitted or dead within a year. Half of surgical discharges are readmitted or dead within a year.

A shocking 81 percent of patients requiring assistance with basic functional needs failed to have a homecare referral, and 64 percent said no one at the hospital talked to them about managing their care at home. The elderly patients, minority patients, patients with low income, or unemployed patients are especially prone to dangerous discharges. It is worth noting that these findings occur more frequently in teaching hospitals than in large community or small hospitals. (2003)

How It Happens

Why are the numbers so startling? Hospital discharge is not a standardized process, and it is just another by-product of discontinuity and fragmentation of care. At this critical time, there is a lack of streamlined communication between multiple doctors and nurses and between them and you. Many people are involved with discharge, increasing the chances of miscommunication. Add to that, many adults have trouble understanding simple health information because of education or literacy issues or dementia.

Little coordination in the "handoff" from the hospital to the rehabilitation facility, to the person assisting you home, or to you directly can also cause issues that lead to poor follow-up care and hospital readmission.

What to Look For

When the big day arrives and you are ready to leave the hospital, slow down and take the time to understand all instructions about your follow-up care. Speak with the social worker, nurse, or discharge administrator to help with the transition. If they are unsure or rushed, ask to have your doctor or a nurse who knows your case attend the meeting.

If you believe you are being discharged before you feel it is safe, talk with your doctor. Sometimes a facility may try to release you because your insurance or Medicare time is about to expire. If this is the case, speak to the hospital discharge planner, your insurance carrier, or the administrator of the hospital. When Mom's Medicare time ran out, one of the insurance coordinators explained they would have to come up with a new complication or diagnosis or move her to another level of care to keep her in the hospital any longer. Because she was in no shape to leave, I told them to do whatever voodoo necessary for her to remain.

Upon discharge, you will receive written discharge instructions. Pay attention to every detail as your discharge nurse reviews them with you. Ask questions if you have any doubts. Bring a list of questions and paper and pen to take notes.

How to Protect Yourself

There is a lot of information to review and questions to ask during discharge, so bring your advocate with you. You may be tired, not feeling well, nervous, and excited to leave, causing you to hurry without asking the correct questions or understanding the given answers. Here are a few key questions:

- Will you need help after you leave the hospital?
- Should someone be with you twenty-four hours a day?
- Will you need home care services, a visiting nurse, or a rehabilitation or skilled nursing home? If so, who will help you navigate your many options?
- Will you need any special equipment at home? If so, has it been prescribed? Where can you get the equipment? Will you have to pick it up or will it be delivered to you? Is it covered by your insurance, Medicare, or other plan?
- How active can you be? Will you need physical therapy? Are there any physical exercises you need to do? If so, get written instructions.
- Are there any restrictions on what you can and cannot do—drive, go back to work, lift, shower, or bathe?
- What signs and symptoms should you watch for?

- If you have drains or wounds, how do you take care of them?
- Will you need to schedule any follow-up visits with your doctor? Will you need to schedule any follow-up tests?
- Get a written list of your medicines and understand when and how to take them and for how long. Are there any foods, vitamins, or drinks that interfere with the medicines?
- What are the potential side effects of all medicines? If so, what should you do if you do experience them?
- Do you know how to reach the doctor 24/7?

The following tips address a few more items that you and your advocate should be capable of performing.

Learn how to monitor any vital signs at home including weight changes, blood pressure, or temperature. If the patient has a drain in place, learn how to empty it and what the fluid from the drain should look like. Also if the patient has a wound, find out who will monitor it. Know how to change dressings if needed.

Keep a written log to track medicines. Write down the dosages and side effects. One of the best drugstore purchases I made was a day-of-the-week plastic pill organizer with long columns of separated boxes. This makes it easy to see if the right pills are taken at the right times. If a pill is forgotten, it is easy to notice because it will still be in the compartment.

Be on the lookout for medicine side effects. A sudden muscle pain may not be a life-threatening situation but instead, a reaction to the medications. Read the pamphlet that comes with the prescriptions. If you have any doubts at all, call the doctor at once. Understand the contraindications of mixing medicines. Some medicines do not play well with others. Learn about any foods or beverages that may interact with prescribed medicines. Any time a new medicine is prescribed, ask the prescriber to review all current medications to check for potential interactions. Your pharmacist can do this for you too.

Check to see if aspirin and other nonsteroidal anti-inflammatory drugs (NSAIDs) are allowed. These products—aspirin, acetaminophen, or combinations of the two (Anacin, Tylenol, Bayer, Excedrin), ibuprofen (Advil, Motrin), and naproxen (Aleve, Naprosyn)—may cause internal bleeding. If you or your patient is taking Coumadin/Warfarin, which is used to prevent blood clots, or other prescription medications—taking NSAIDs may increase the risk of internal bleeding. Beware of combination products. NyQuil and other cough and cold remedies are combination products that also contain NSAID ingredients. Do not assume that over-the-counter medications are safe just because they are over the counter. This includes nutritional supplements, herbs, and teas. To avoid any dangerous interactions, always ask the doctor and pharmacist before you or your patient self-prescribe.

Understand the dietary restrictions you or your patient may have. This is not a matter to take lightly. A restricted diet is not fun and games like a weight loss diet before a big date or party. Visitors never seem to take this seriously. "Oh, have another chip. It won't hurt you," might be okay if you are trying to lose a pound or two; however, it is not safe if you are on a no-salt diet.

Mom was on a no-salt diet in an attempt to control her volume overload. Volume overload occurs when there is too much fluid in the blood. In Mom's case this was caused by hospital acquired congestive heart failure and subsequent excessive sodium intake. The excess fluid, made up of salt and water, built up in her system. This led to an increase in weight, swelling in the legs and arms, and fluid in her abdomen. Gradually, the fluid entered the air spaces surrounding her lungs, reducing the amount of oxygen that enters the blood, causing shortness of breath.

Each day her weight inched higher and higher. The diuretic pills (water pills) did little to lessen the fluid buildup. The doctors resorted to a last-chance procedure called aquapheresis. Using catheters, the process withdraws blood, and then passes the blood through a special filter. The filter separates the excess salt and water from the blood. The blood is returned to the body through a continuous loop, while the excess fluid collects in a bag for measurement and disposal.

Over the course of several days, the procedure withdrew over thirty pounds of fluid from her body. In the meantime, she continued to eat the food delivered to her room. In less than a week, the fluid built up again, and we watched her weight increase, her legs and feet swell, and her breathing become labored. No one seemed to understand why this was happening. What was causing the continual fluid buildup?

One evening as Mom circled blueberry muffins and butter on her breakfast menu, I looked at her choices. The menu, titled "cardiac diet," was a "lower" sodium diet of 1500 mg of salt per day. She needed a "no-salt" diet to assist with lessening the fluid buildup in her body. Unknowingly, we were fighting against ourselves, as the dieticians sent salted foods while the doctors drained fluid caused by salt. Although I brought this to everyone's attention, nothing much changed. So I self-imposed the changes by bringing in no-salt foods and monitoring Mom's hospital menu choices. For days, the kitchen sent salted butter even though I requested no-salt butter. It was just another one of my "I can't believe this" daily struggles.

As soon as I brought Mom home, I served foods with no salt at all, in an extreme effort to get rid of the fluid. Although she kicked and screamed—the daily weigh-ins proved my course of action was justified. When the fluid weight dropped and leveled, I gradually added a little more salt to her diet. Today, with her good management, she enjoys most of her usual foods, and her weight remains at a safe level.

This story illustrates the need for an advocate—to act as a patient's radar—to watch for every grain of salt while in the hospital or out. If you are the advocate and your patient is disagreeable, help him or her understand the ramifications of noncompliance. Supply reading material that attests to your reasoning. Stay steadfast in what is in the best interests of your patient.

Going home should be a time to get better and get on with your life. It is the goal of your hospital stay. By paying strict attention to discharge instructions and tending to follow-up, you can put the hospital on your list of never events.

Medical Risks That Should Never Happen

Many of the risks discussed in this chapter are included in Medicare's list of *Never Events*. Even if you are not a Medicare patient, the Centers for Medicare & Medicaid Services (CMS) Never Events affect you. The policy addresses events that should never happen during a hospital stay. The CMS announced they would no longer pay for additional costs associated with many preventable errors, including those considered Never Events. If a Never Event takes place, you will not have to pay to address the error. The additional expense now falls on the responsible hospital.

To round out your knowledge of hospital hazards, I am including several medical errors considered by CMS as Never Events.

Surgical Events

- Surgery or other invasive procedure performed on the wrong site or the wrong patient
- Unintended retention of a foreign object in a patient after surgery or other invasive procedure

Product or Device Events

- Patient death or serious injury associated with the use of contaminated drugs, devices, or biologics provided by the health care setting

Patient Protection Events

- Patient suicide, attempted suicide, or self-harm that results in serious injury while being cared for in a health care setting

Care Management Events

- Patient death or serious injury associated with a medication error (e.g., errors involving the wrong drug, wrong dose, wrong patient, wrong time, wrong rate, wrong preparation, or wrong route of administration)
- Patient death or serious injury associated with unsafe administration of blood products
- Patient death or serious injury associated with a fall while being cared for in a health care setting
- Any stage 3, stage 4, and unstageable pressure ulcers acquired after admission/presentation to a health care setting
- Patient death or serious injury resulting from failure to follow

up or communicate laboratory, pathology, or radiology test
results

Environmental Events

- Any incident in which systems designated for oxygen or other
  gas to be delivered to a patient contains no gas, the wrong gas,
  or is contaminated by toxic substances
- Radiologic events
- Death or serious injury of a patient or staff associated with the
  introduction of a metallic object into the MRI area

Potential Criminal Events

- Abduction of a patient/resident of any age
- Death or serious injury of a patient or staff member resulting
  from a physical assault (i.e., battery) that occurs in or on the
  grounds of a health care setting

For more information about Never Events, visit CMS's website
(www.cms.gov).

Almost every hospital hazard hinges on judgment and human
error. Because doctors and nurses have diverse experiences, education,
cultures, personality, and emotional and spiritual differences, you can
expect each person to view your situation with a different attitude and
opinion. Although this diversity gives you choices and options, it also
creates space for judgment calls. Whom do you trust to make the final
call? Will that call be an error? All you can do is be educated, perceptive
and willing to speak up.

CHAPTER 7

Other Ominous Encounters

MANY risks are inherent throughout a hospital stay. A few make the news; others go unmentioned. It is difficult to discuss all of the possible dangers in the scope of one book. However I did encounter the following during Mom's adventure and I find them worthy of mention.

Suicide

In a follow-up report on preventing suicide titled *Focus on medical/ surgical units and the emergency department*, the Joint Commission says,

> Hospital suicide is one of the top five most frequently reported events to The Joint Commission. Men take their lives at nearly four times the rate as women, and men ages seventy-five and older have the highest rate of suicide. Hospitalized patients are three times more likely to attempt suicide than nonhospitalized patients.
>
> While psychiatric settings are designed to be safe for suicidal individuals and have staff with specialized training, typically, medical/surgical units and emergency departments are not designed or assessed for suicide risk and do not have staff with specialized training to deal with suicidal individuals...It is note-worthy that many patients who kill themselves in general hospital inpatient units do not have a psychiatric history or a history of suicide attempt. Compared to the psychiatric hospital and unit, the general hospital setting also presents more access to items

that can be used to attempt suicide – items that are either already in or may be brought into the facility and more opportunities for the patient to be alone to attempt or re-attempt suicide…

The risk factors common across health care settings include a recent suicide attempt, suicidal thoughts or behaviors, a family history of suicide or psychiatric illness. The use of medications such as antidepressants, physical health problems, diagnosis of delirium or dementia, chronic pain, poor prognosis or prospect of certain death can be contributing factors. Social stressors such as financial strain, unemployment, disability, divorce or other relationship problems are triggers. Substance abuse may also exacerbate depression and other psychological symptoms, and the effects of alcohol may contribute to impulsive suicidal behavior. Older adults are prone to additional suicide risk factors including declining health, loneliness and recent bereavement.

Warning signs associated with imminent risk include irrita-bility, increased anxiety, panic, agitation, impulsivity, decreased emotional reactivity, complaining of unrelenting pain, refusing visitors, crying spells, declining medications and requesting early discharge. In addition, the following warning signs are diagnostic criteria for depression: hopelessness or helplessness, decreased interest in treatment or prognosis, feelings of worth-lessness, and refusing to eat.

There are numerous medications associated with an increased risk of suicidal thoughts and behaviors, including antide-pressants, anti-epileptic or anticonvulsant medicines, and anti-psychotic agents. The risk of suicidal thoughts and behav-iors applies to both psychiatric and non-psychiatric uses of these medications. Certain other medicines have also been associated with increased risk of suicide, such as some smoking-cessation drugs and anti-infectives. (2010)

When the doctors gave Mom psychotropic drugs to assist with her supposed depression, she became increasingly more depressed. She experienced drug-induced delirium, had frequent hallucinations, and became irritable thanks to the drugs BuSpar, Sertraline, and a host of others. Sertraline carries a black box warning that states, "Patients of all ages who are started on therapy should be monitored appropriately and observed closely for clinical worsening, suicidality or unusual changes in behavior" and "close observation for suicidal thinking."

Many times, these drug-induced psychiatric reactions caused her to ask me to cover her face with the pillow. In her messed-up mind, she'd had enough. As an advocate, I put an end to the unwarranted use of these drugs, and soon she came back to reality. She thanks me today for not honoring her requests. Advocates should monitor drugs and their side effects. Ask if it is safe to reduce the dose or eliminate the use of risky medications.

The need for a round-the-clock advocate is imperative if the patient has any suicide risk inclinations or if he or she takes any medications with risky mind-altering side effects. If you have any doubts or concerns, ask for a suicide or mental health risk assessment. Ask the staff to check the patient and room for suicide-assisting goods or devices including call light cords, IV tubing, plastic bags, belts, shoelaces, or razors. During handoff times (when patient care is transferred from doctor to doctor, nurse to nurse, shift to shift, and location to location) alert all hospital staff of any warning signs or suicide risks, as this is a prime opportunity for miscommunication. Upon the patient's discharge from the hospital, be sure to get appropriate follow-up information and instructions.

Additional Suicide Prevention Resources

- The American Foundation for Suicide Prevention (www.afsp.org)
- National Suicide Prevention Lifeline (www.suicideprevention-lifeline.org or 1-800-273-TALK (8255))
- The Veterans Crisis Line (www.veteranscrisisline.net) or 1-800-273-8255

Diabetes

My first encounter with diabetes was during Mom's hospital stay. She never had diabetes before surgery, and pre-admission blood tests did not indicate a problem. However, during the weeks of her stay in ICU, there was talk about diabetes. Each day the staff took glucose tests with fingersticks, and each morning gave Mom a shot of insulin in her abdomen. At the time I did not understand why she was suddenly diabetic. One of the nurses who came to be a friend gave me a lesson.

Diabetes is a metabolic disorder that alters the way the body uses digested food for energy and growth. Your body turns food into a sugar called glucose. The bloodstream carries glucose to your cells. Insulin, a hormone produced by the pancreas, helps glucose enter your cells where it turns into energy. If your body does not make enough insulin or if the released insulin cannot do its job, the glucose builds up in the bloodstream. This causes high blood glucose levels or hyperglycemia. Complications from high blood sugar include increased risk of heart attacks, strokes, kidney failure, loss of eyesight, and limb amputation.

Normal blood glucose or sugar levels are 70–99 mg/dL when fasting and before meals. The normal levels after meals are 70—140 mg/dL. Blood sugar levels do not have to be extremely high for hyperglycemia to be dangerous. Blood sugar levels consistently near 150 mg/ dL can be dangerous, possibly resulting in sepsis—an illness where the blood-stream is flooded with bacteria.

The types of diabetes are:

- Type 1 diabetes (previously known as juvenile onset diabetes)
- Type 2 diabetes (previously known as adult onset diabetes)
- Gestational diabetes (occurs during pregnancy)
- Hospital-, stress-, or medicine-induced hyperglycemia

Hospital-induced hyperglycemia can develop because of stress or medications. Stress-induced hyperglycemia is the elevation of the blood glucose caused by the stress of an illness, surgery, or anesthesia.

Medicine-induced diabetes is the result of certain drugs that prevent insulin from working, causing high or sometimes low blood sugar levels.

Many patients who exhibit high blood sugar during their hospital stays have no prior history of diabetes. The hospital setting is the first clue to early diabetes. This makes screening tests very important upon hospital admission (they serve as a baseline) as well as continued monitoring throughout a hospital stay. Even mildly elevated blood sugar levels can increase morbidity and mortality. So, it is essential to identify hyperglycemia at the time of hospital admission and to initiate means to maintain normal levels, regardless of your primary reason for admission or previous diabetes status.

In Mom's case, not only did she withstand high-stress emergency heart surgeries—she also had to deal with ingesting almost every category of drug known to elevate blood sugar levels. This newly acquired problem was a common result that came as a surprise to me.

Hospital-induced hyperglycemia has the same outcomes as diabetes and warrants the same treatment. Patients with untreated hyperglycemia have a higher risk of infection, return to surgery more often, and experience other serious complications—wound, bloodstream, and other hospital-acquired infections; cardiac arrhythmia; acute renal failure; blood transfusions; ventilator support; and urinary tract infections. Diabetes can also double your risk of heart attack and stroke.

Many medications cause high glucose levels. Levels may resume to normal once you eliminate the offending drugs. Fortunately, this was the case for my mom. However, you may need to monitor your levels even after you discontinue those drugs. Drugs to watch out for are steroids, diuretics or water pills, beta-blockers, antipsychotic medications, estrogen, antibiotics, and chemotherapy drugs.

Steroids cause an increase in blood sugar, especially in people with diabetes, by blocking the release of insulin. Hydrocortisone and prednisone used to treat symptoms associated with respiratory disorders or inflammatory diseases can also increase blood sugar levels.

Diuretics, or water pills, act on the kidneys to cause increased urine output to remove excess fluid from the body. Many diuretics, particularly thiazide and furosemide, have the potential to cause hyperglycemia. Diuretics lower the levels of potassium in the blood and lead to decreased release of insulin by the pancreas—the organ responsible for lowering blood sugar. If you take diuretics, inquire about supplemental potassium. Ask for a blood test to monitor your potassium levels.

Beta-blockers including metoprolol, propanolol, and atenolol, among others, serve to decrease the heart rate or blood pressure and treat angina and heart failure. Beta-blockers can increase blood sugar in diabetic and nondiabetic patients, and push a borderline diabetic into type 2 diabetes. Antipsychotic medications, namely lithium, olanzapine, and risperidone are responsible for increasing blood sugars. Monitor the use of these drugs closely.

The female hormone estrogen, when taken as an oral contraceptive or as a supplement for menopause, has the ability to raise blood sugar levels as well. The antibiotic, gatifloxacin, a member of the fluoroquinolone family, can cause either high or low blood sugar levels in both diabetics and nondiabetics.

The chemotherapy drug bortezomib, used to treat blood and bone marrow cancers, may cause a rise in blood sugar levels. All patients receiving chemotherapy should monitor their blood sugar levels. Other drugs known to alter blood sugar levels are azathioprine, used to treat rheumatoid arthritis; protease inhibitors, used as HIV and cancer treatments; in addition to certain calcium channel blockers and the stomach antacid cimetidine, better known as Tagamet, used to treat ulcers or the symptoms of gastroesophageal reflux disease (GERD).

Diabetes often goes undiagnosed because many of its symptoms seem harmless. Early detection of diabetes symptoms and treatment can decrease the chance of developing the complications of diabetes. If you are in the hospital or not, these are the warning signs:

- *Type 1 diabetes*—frequent urination, unusual thirst, extreme hunger, unusual weight loss, extreme fatigue, and irritability.
- *Type 2 diabetes*—any of the type 1 symptoms, frequent infections, blurred vision, cuts/bruises that are slow to heal, tingling/numbness in the hands/feet, and gum or bladder infections. (Often, people with type 2 diabetes have no symptoms.)

Diabetes is the fourth most common comorbidity encountered in hospitals, meaning it shows up in addition to your main medical problem. Elevated sugar levels are associated with poor hospital outcomes and can predict mortality in heart attack or MI patients with and without diabetes. If you or a loved one must stay in the hospital, ask for a simple blood test to screen for elevated blood sugar levels. Throughout your hospital stay, be sure someone monitors your levels. Ask for the results, and keep track of them. If your levels rise beyond normal limits, ask for appropriate treatment.

The Centers for Disease Control and Prevention (CDC) has become increasingly concerned about the risks for transmitting hepatitis B virus (HBV) and other infectious diseases during assisted blood glucose (blood sugar) monitoring and insulin administration. In a paper titled, Infection Prevention during Blood Glucose Monitoring and Insulin Administration, they summarize:

An under appreciated risk of blood glucose testing is the opportunity for exposure to blood borne viruses (HBV, hepatitis C virus, and HIV) through contaminated equipment and supplies if devices used for testing and/or insulin administration (e.g., blood glucose meters, fingerstick devices, insulin pens) are shared.

Outbreaks of hepatitis B virus (HBV) infection associated with blood glucose monitoring have been identified with increasing regularity, particularly in long-term care settings, such as nursing homes and assisted living facilities, where residents often require assistance with monitoring of blood glucose levels and/or insulin administration. In the last 10 years, at least 15 outbreaks of HBV infection are associated with providers failing to follow basic principles of infection control when assisting with blood glucose monitoring. Because of under-reporting and under recognition, the number of outbreaks due to unsafe diabetes care practices identified to date are likely an underestimate. Although the majority of these outbreaks have been reported in long-term care settings, the risk of infection is present in any setting where blood glucose monitoring equipment is shared or those assisting with blood glucose monitoring and/or insulin administration fail to follow basic principles of infection control. Recently, at a health fair in New Mexico in 2010, dozens of attendees were potentially exposed to blood borne viruses when fingerstick devices were inappropriately reused for multiple persons to conduct diabetes screening. Additionally, at a hospital in Texas in 2009, more than 2,000 persons were notified and recommended to undergo testing for blood borne viruses after individual insulin pens were used for multiple persons. (2011)

Before every blood sugar monitoring or insulin administration, remind your health care provider to wash his or her hands, wear new gloves, and disinfect the blood glucose meter. Always use a new fingerstick device or insulin pen.

For more information on diabetes, visit the American Diabetes Association website (www.diabetes.org).

Therapy

"Physical therapy starts at eleven every weekday in the therapy room down the hall." A nurse's aide mentioned this as Mom checked in to the rehabilitation center. Little did I know that the next six weeks would be the most stressful part of our journey. Mom was extremely weak and could not walk. Diagnosed with heart failure; hooked to a urine catheter, an oxygen tank, multiple IVs, and a nasogastric feeding tube; and burdened with a stage four bedsore and an immobilized shoulder, she needed professional assistance for even the simplest of tasks. The only way to move her involved two people and a Hoyer lift—a hydraulic sling that carried her from bed to wheelchair.

There were many tasks involved to prepare for her 11:00 AM therapy appointment. She had to eat breakfast, take medications, talk with the doctors during their rounds, have the wound team clean and bandage the bedsore, go to the bathroom, get a bed bath, change clothes, unhook oxygen and other IVs, get lifted from the bed to the wheelchair, rehook oxygen and IVs, get weighed, and get wheeled to therapy. This was a lot to accomplish for a sick patient who relied on others for help.

During our first week, I counted on the staff to get Mom to therapy on time. I figured they knew the routine. I was wrong. Mom never made it to therapy that week. By the time the staff showed up to get her ready, the therapists had gone elsewhere for lunch. Without physical and occupational therapy, Mom would not regain her ability to walk, dress, or feed herself. I realized that in order for her to get to therapy on time, we had to start around 9:00 AM. Each day after breakfast, medications, and doctor visits, I had to call for an aide as a reminder to give Mom a bath and change her clothes. Usually an hour passed before someone helped.

Invariably, after the bath, we had to call for a bedpan. This took another twenty minutes and a lot of me standing outside her door with hands on my hips to get someone to respond. Then we endured the daily game of hide-and-seek with the Hoyer lift. It was never on the floor, so someone had to run around in an attempt to locate it. Once it was found, it took about thirty minutes to unravel all of the IV tubes, position the sling, and hoist Mom from bed to chair. This was an exhausting ordeal for her and usually called for another fifteen minutes of rest and oxygen.

The therapist was supposed to arrive at the room at 10:55 AM to wheel Mom to therapy; he usually arrived twenty minutes later. As her advocate, I hooked the oxygen tank to the wheelchair and took her to therapy on time by myself. The frenzied preparation and mom's fragile health caused her to arrive at therapy in utter fatigue. She did her best to attempt the tasks assigned yet apparently not as well as the therapist expected. Behind our backs, he spoke with Mom's doctors and suggested antidepressants. He believed Mom was holding back from fear and deemed the antipsychotic drugs would cause her to progress at his pace.

The rehabilitation center employed an ever-changing team of hospitalists. Each week Mom had a different doctor with different methods. Each doctor tried to outsmart the previous doctor, and so began our Baskin-Robbins antipsychotic drug flavor of the week nightmare. During the next five weeks, Mom was not her normal self. She saw people standing behind her and babies on the dresser; had bizarre and frightening dreams; and ironically was incapable of concentrating on therapy. Meanwhile, I struggled with the morning routine, begging, cajoling, and pleading with the nurses to respond in a timely manner so we could get to therapy. I finally fired all of the doctors except for one and he slowly weaned Mom from the offensive drugs.

Throughout all of this, she experienced extreme fluid overload. Her weight skyrocketed, and she had trouble breathing. Shockingly, no doctor or nurse said or did anything about this. One afternoon, a young RN pulled me aside and said, "You need to get your mom out of here and into the hospital today." Then she taught me how to use a stethoscope. "Listen to the sounds as she breathes." I heard clicking, rattling, and crackling noises made by Mom's lungs, indicating pneumonia or pulmonary edema. In a few hours I checked her back into the intensive care unit.

The physical therapy situation did not improve in the hospital. Although the doctors performed miraculous medical feats, the therapy staff lagged behind. My goal was to get Mom out of the hospital and back home. Each day in the hospital increased the potential for infection or other mismanaged event. During the first week, a physical therapist came by the room to get Mom out of bed to walk. He brought a big rolling walker with him. She walked a few steps and quickly ran out of breath. Back in bed, the therapist had her move her fingers and wrists. This too was a struggle. As he left the room, he said, "I'll be back tomorrow and we will do this again." Tomorrow came and went and so did the rest of the week. No therapist, no walking, and no mention of therapy by any of the nurses.

Once again, as an advocate, I questioned the nurses each day, "Is someone going to walk with my mom today?" They rolled their eyes in sympathy as I told the tale of the missing therapist. They had seen it many times with other patients, so occasionally a kind nurse stopped her daily routine to help Mom walk. I made a lot of noise about this to our doctors and the staff. "How are we supposed to get out of here if she cannot walk, dress, bathe, or eat by herself?" It was a constant struggle that did not resolve itself on this floor.

Once her cardiac events were under control, the hospital discharged Mom back to the former rehabilitation center. Again, as an advocate I fought against that. Going back there would be similar to playing with a boomerang. I feared spending the rest of Mom's life bouncing from rehab to the hospital and back. I had to find a place where people took therapy seriously. After scores of conversations and visits to facilities, I found one. At this location, Mom's physical therapist helped her walk and taught her how to use her new shoulder. An occupational therapist helped her regain the movements needed to perform the activities of normal daily living. In three weeks, Mom was walking unattended with a walker, eating with utensils, climbing stairs, and playing Wii bowling games. The afternoon I watched her make cookies with her therapist, I wept uncontrollably. I never thought I would see that day.

If ever there was a need for an advocate, it was then. No one took her therapy seriously. No one followed up. There was no continuity, no procedures, and no rules. The situation forced me to behave as a crazy person—calling, ringing, waiting, huffing, and asking, "What good is tricky heart surgery if she cannot regain mobility? Why aren't stringent therapy procedures in place? How is she supposed to walk out of the hospital if she cannot walk?"

In return, I got shrugs and blank stares. My mom was in no shape physically, mentally, or emotionally to struggle with the tracking down of therapists or timely therapy. The staff was not attentive. Only an advocate with the willingness to follow through could navigate through the indifference. If you find yourself in the position of needing physical or occupational therapy while in the hospital, be mindful of the pitfalls. If you are an advocate, set the stage on the very first day that you expect therapy on a regular basis. If this does not happen—speak up. And speak up again and again until you achieve results.

CHAPTER 8

The Senior Scenario

THE elderly are at a great risk for hospital-induced conditions. The Department of Health and Human Services reports, "Of the nearly 1 million Medicare beneficiaries discharged from hospitals in October 2008, about one in seven experienced an adverse event" (2010). Many issues can complicate recovery or set off an entirely new chain reaction of medical issues—drug reactions, pressure sores, falls, continence issues, dehydration, nutritional concerns, difficulty with pain or sleep, hospital-induced delirium, dementia, miscommunication at discharge, end-of-life decision making, and newly acquired functional limitations.

Elective surgery poses added exposure for heart attacks and strokes for the senior population. Presurgical testing, consultations, and risk assessments with a geriatric specialist need to be thorough. Early diagnosis is difficult in elderly people. It is easy to ignore symptoms and attribute them to "old age." Left unchecked, a disease can take hold until it is too advanced to handle.

Socioeconomic issues come in to play as well. Many seniors live alone and have financial constraints with no one to depend on. They suffer in silence until a health care issue becomes painfully obvious. Older women are especially at risk because of longevity factors. Many senior women also live alone and struggle to care for themselves. The need for an advocate to act in conjunction with or for an older person is paramount.

Adverse Drug Reactions

Seniors experience adverse drug reactions because of physical changes brought on by age that affect how the body handles drugs. Seniors also see numerous physicians, use more prescription drugs, and fill their prescriptions at different pharmacies.

Older patients may receive one or more medications from their primary care physician and additional medications from specialty physicians without each other's knowledge. As seniors see more physicians, even more medications are prescribed, increasing the chance of a risky combination. Because the average senior receives 25 prescriptions each year, they are four times more likely to be hospitalized due to an ADR. Sadly, over three-fourths of cases are found to be preventable. One study found that one out of four older adults was prescribed a "potentially inappropriate" drug or drugs, placing them at risk for adverse drug effects.

Not only can a drug prescription be inappropriate; combinations of drugs can also be problematic, and the duration of treatment can be too long and unsafe. In a paper titled *Interactions Cause Seniors to Drop Antidepressants*, Reuters Health Information stated, "We found a concerning degree of potentially harmful drug combinations being prescribed to seniors. Older adults are often taking dangerous combinations of prescription drugs, but doctors are not getting the message" (2010).

In addition, a few classes of drugs are known to be major sources of ADRs. Many older adults currently take one of the following of these drug classes: cardiovascular drugs, cancer drugs, psychotropic drugs, namely tranquilizers and antidepressants, and anti-inflammatory drugs. The inability to maintain a healthy blood pressure is common in older adults and is further hampered by the use of these kinds of drugs. In addition, tranquilizers, antidepressants, antipsychotic drugs, antihistamines, or drugs for heart conditions can cause dizziness upon standing or getting out of bed, increasing the risk for falls.

Many adults become thin and frail as they age. The normal dosage of medications may be too high for the smaller body to handle, causing unanticipated reactions. A large proportion of medications are processed through the liver and kidneys. Older people with decreased organ function do not have the capacity to clear drugs from their systems. The combination of smaller body weight and decreased organ function allows drugs to accumulate in the body at high levels for long periods. This can cause damage.

Drugs that act on the central nervous system—sleeping pills, tranquilizers, antidepressants, antipsychotic drugs, and antihistamines, are called *anticholinergic*. Older adults have an extra sensitivity to these drugs and should not use them unless needed. In addition to a host of physical side effects, the mental effects—including delirium, confusion, and memory problems—can rapidly change the quality of life for the patient and the family.

Older adults or those prone to anxiety issues should avoid stimulant drugs because they can cause dangerous effects on blood pressure and heart function. Drugs used for nasal and sinus decongestants contain the stimulant pseudoephedrine, a member of the amphetamine class of drugs. Prescription drugs aren't the only drugs that can cause issues for seniors. Sudafed, Claritin-D, Zyrtec, and other outwardly innocuous over-the-counter medications contain dangerous ingredients for sensitive seniors.

It helps to realize the serious differences between a young person's ability to handle a drug and an older person's ability to handle the same drug. Older adults are less able to compensate for potential side effects. The variables used to determine the level of risk of an ADR in an older adult are—the number of medications used, the number of medical conditions, any previous adverse reactions, and the existence of heart or kidney failure or liver disease. Because the number of medications is the strongest predictor of risk, always ask about the following information and keep track of it in your safety log: drug name, drug class, dosage amount, duration of treatment, and the known and potential side effects. By increasing your awareness, you may be able to take fewer drugs in lower doses and experience fewer effects.

Drug- or hospital-induced delirium, sometimes called ICU psychosis, can be caused by the combination of drugs, sleep deprivation, pain, dehydration, and the disturbance of the body's natural rhythm. The use of antipsychotics, sedatives, or antidepressants can actually worsen the situation. According to estimates, a whopping 80 percent of elderly intensive care patients develop delirium. I watched it happen to Mom during her hospital stay and I adamantly insisted upon the halt of all antidepressants.

If you are an advocate, especially for a patient in ICU or a patient who has a lengthy hospital stay, be aware of the signs of delirium and take steps to avoid it. Do not allow a new medication to start or an old medication to stop without your knowledge. Be on the lookout for slurred speech or crazy-looking eyes, agitation, depression, hallucinations, confusion, memory loss, strange storytelling, or anything else that doesn't "seem right."

Take the following steps to bypass the triggers that, when combined with drugs, can create an atmosphere for mental confusion and disorientation:

- Try to reduce or eliminate drugs known to encourage mental changes.
- Have an advocate in the room at all times to monitor changes. An advocate can offer familiarity and stability in an otherwise frightening sea of strangers.
- Keep visits with family and friends quiet and calm, and avoid stressful conversations or arguments.
- Make sure the patient is well hydrated. Dehydration can contribute to confusion.
- Keep a large clock and calendar nearby. Each morning, remind the patient of the day of the week, the date, and year.
- To prevent disorientation, keep eyeglasses or hearing aids in reach.
- Be aware of "sundowning"—a disruption of the body's "internal clock" that occurs during the late afternoon and involves unusually agitated or disoriented behavior.

To prevent sundowning in particular, coordinate lighting with day and night and allow dark and uninterrupted sleep at night. If the room has a window, open the blinds in the daytime to allow natural light to enter the room. Close the blinds at sunset to keep the room dark. Ask the staff not to wake the patient in the middle of the night to do things they can easily do during the day. At Mom's rehabilitation center, the night staff routinely gave her a bed bath at 3:30 AM—presumably to lessen their workload during the day. Once again, as her advocate, I had to speak up and say, "No."

Deleterious Discharges

Older adults have a high hospital readmission rate. In fact, an article in the New England Journal of Medicine called, *Rehospitalizations among patients in the Medicare fee-for-service program* reveals, "35 percent of Medicare patients are readmitted within ninety days of discharge" (2009). This is largely because the discharge process is fragmented and flawed to begin with, and many seniors have elderly spouses, friends, or perhaps no one to help decipher and fulfill the cryptic discharge instructions. Medical information can be misunderstood, prescriptions not filled, and in-home plans of action not followed. The family caregivers of those with multiple medical conditions and multiple drug requirements may also be elderly, sick, or too frail to assist with the follow-up.

Most readmissions are linked to lack of follow-up care. Many older patients need help with the activities of daily living after a hospital stay. For those who live alone, the rate for readmission doubles from those who have help at home.

The loss of mental acuity, vision, or hearing impairment can also contribute to diagnosis and treatment misunderstandings both during the hospital stay and at discharge. For these reasons and many others, seniors have a great need for a patient advocate.

Tracey Driscoll, RN, MHA advocates for seniors via her company, Transition with Care, in Concord, Massachusetts. She understands the vulnerable space between discharge and home. She says,

> Change is stressful for everyone, but for older adults, it can be particularly difficult. How to navigate the next step can seem even more overwhelming. Seniors need help to promote independence at home. Prior to discharge, we perform a personalized audit of home safety and activities of daily living requirements. Then we offer specific recommendations to address individual needs and safety concerns including home modifications, referrals for community services, in-home healthcare services and

procurement of healthcare equipment, supplies and resources as needed. To provide continuity, we monitor the elder's care through regularly scheduled and documented visits and communicate with family via written reports, e-mail and telephone. (Driscoll, pers. comm.)

To ensure a safe discharge, senior patients should always have a capable family member, friend, or advocate attend the discharge meeting. Get written discharge instructions. Ask for a risk of fall assessment and a frailty assessment before going home.

During the meeting, your advocate should take notes about medication management. Discharge is a prime occasion for medication mix-ups. Old prescriptions, lingering in bathroom drawers at home may no longer be appropriate. New prescriptions may need to be filled. Start a new log to include all current medication names, dosages, and side effects. Write down the reason for your admission, procedures done, and the outcomes. Do you have any follow-up appointments, therapy plans, and arrangements for home care? Next find out what activities you may and may not do. What signs or symptoms should you question?

Then ensure your home environment will accommodate post-hospital needs. Do you need any medical equipment; oxygen, a walker, a wheelchair, or a special bed? If so, how will you get these items? Does someone need to stay with you at home? When and for how long? Do you have the people in place, or do you need help with this?

Medicare may cover nursing services, physical therapy, and other services. Use the hospital's discharge planner as a resource and guide to help with your *safe* transition home.

Seniors Still at Risk

The last time the United States assessed the risks of hospitals was in 1999. At that time, the Institute of Medicine released a report titled, *To Err is Human, Building a Safer Health System* and found that up to 98,000 patients died each year from medical mistakes (1999). The following is an excerpt from the most recent report from the Department of Health and Human Services, titled *Adverse events in hospitals: National incidence among Medicare beneficiaries*:

In the decade since the 1999 Institute of Medicine report, the need to improve patient safety has received much attention from Federal and State governments, advocacy groups, and the health care industry. Despite this attention, we found that 13.5 percent of Medicare beneficiaries experienced adverse events during their hospital stays in October 2008, most of which resulted in prolonged hospital stays, permanent harm, life-sustaining interventions, or death. Of the nearly 1 million Medicare beneficiaries discharged from hospitals in October 2008, about one in seven experienced an adverse event that met at least one of our criteria (13.5 percent). This rate projects to an estimated 134,000 Medicare beneficiaries experiencing at least one adverse event in hospitals during the 1-month study period. An additional 13.5 percent of beneficiaries experienced temporary harm as the result of events. Additionally, 28 percent of beneficiaries who experienced adverse events also had temporary harm events during the same stay. Physician reviewers determined that 44 percent of events were preventable and that preventable events often involved medical errors, substandard care, and inadequate monitoring or assessment of patients. We found that in addition to causing the harm to patients, adverse events and temporary harm events increased costs to Medicare by an estimated $324 million in a single month (2010).

Senior Advocacy

Because one in seven seniors still experience a preventable adverse medical event, it is important to understand that senior patients may not have the awareness, capability, or strength to watch for signs of hospital risks. Pressure sores are prevalent because of thinner skin, malnutrition, and not being mindful enough to move and rotate positions. Adverse drug reactions occur with great frequency in older patients. Hospital falls are common. In addition to these physical ramifications, older patients deal with loss of decision-making control. Elderly spouses or adult children with their own biases must often step in to make medical judgment calls or plan for new living arrangements. End-of-life decisions may have to be determined.

Hospitalized seniors have special needs that transcend the scope of pure medicine. The presence of an advocate is crucial at this time of life. Even if the patient has supportive friends and relatives, sometimes the entire family network needs help and guidance. Sometimes it is wise to call on an outside professional trained to recognize and handle these individual needs.

Barbara Abruzzo RN, founder and owner of Livingwell Care Navigation Inc. New York, New York, says,

> Healthcare professionals often focus solely on the physical manifestations of an illness and ignore the emotional and spiritual components. This limited focus on symptom management often leads to a lack of overall quality of life that people desire. For consumers dealing with an ill, aging, or dying parent or loved one, support for the challenges, such as choosing a facility, signing a do not resuscitate order, or dealing with one's own emotional turmoil around those decisions is often lacking. Healthcare navigation specialists are trained to support the whole person on a physical, emotional, and spiritual level. Our goal is to assure that our clients understand the totality of their own needs, and are supported on all levels to achieve the highest quality of life attainable. (Abruzzo. pers. comm.)

The elderly need extra attention when faced with a hospital stay. Ideally, the hospital should be responsible for a successful outcome. In reality, older patients need an advocate—a family member, friend, or a hired professional—to make sure their needs are met.

CHAPTER 9

Warnings for Women

WOMEN have special health care issues that require particular attention. The many differences between the health care needs of women and men, and the documented disparities in health care between the two, are evident. Heart attack warning signs go unrecognized, labor and delivery are mishandled, and endometriosis is dismissed as a normal period.

Many potential hospital issues begin at the doctor's office. A hospital stay may be avoided if diagnoses and treatments are handled correctly at an early point of an illness. Yet many women's health issues present themselves with deceitful symptoms, making it easy for a doctor to render a false diagnosis. That is why it is imperative for women to educate themselves before they have symptoms.

Major issues involving women's health include the following:

- breast cancer and other cancers
- mammography
- reproductive health and organ diseases
- menstruation and premenstrual syndromes
- contraception and family planning issues
- fertility/infertility issues
- menopause issues and hormone replacement therapy
- heart health
- pregnancy, prenatal care, miscarriage and postpartum depression

Cancers

A late diagnosis or misdiagnosis of cancer can mean the difference between life and death. Many cancers can be treated if the symptoms are recognized and treatment begins early.

Breast Cancer

Mammograms or manual breast exams usually identify breast cancer. However, despite diligent patient care, breast cancer may be missed. Mammograms may be misread. False negatives and false positives can lead to unnecessary surgery and other invasive procedures or to a clear report when in fact a problem exists. A breast lump can be missed during a routine OB-GYN visit because of a less-than-thorough exam. This can lead to a failure to recommend a follow-up mammogram, a failure to biopsy any suspicious lumps, or a failure to follow up with an oncologist. Also, an incorrect staging of breast cancer can lead to overly aggressive or too few treatments.

Cervical Cancer

Cervical cancer may be diagnosed after a Pap smear, biopsy, or other test. Many times Pap smears come back with inconclusive results, classify a normal smear as suspicious or fail to detect abnormal cells. Laboratory errors can cause abnormal results due to sample contamination.

Pap smears are often analyzed incorrectly. False negatives, which are more common than false positives, frequently occur. Inadequate sampling and improper slide preparation may be responsible for most of all false negatives or failure to recognize or correctly classify abnormal cells.

Because Pap test samples usually travel from a doctor's office to a laboratory, a sample can become compromised in many ways. If the sample is not packaged properly, it could be exposed to heat and moisture. If the sample is dropped, it could become contaminated and cause abnormal results. If you have any doubt as to the accuracy of your Pap test, request an immediate repeat. Ask your doctor how you will be notified of the results. Insist on a phone call and a written report, regardless of the results. Keep the results in your medical file.

Remember, an abnormal pap test never leads directly to treatment, and it is not a diagnosis. A diagnosis is made by a colposcopy and biopsy. Only upon these exam findings should a treatment be advised. If a hysterectomy is suggested because of an abnormal Pap test, get additional opinions.

Ovarian Cancer

The American Cancer Society estimates that almost 22,000 women in the United States will be diagnosed with ovarian cancer each year, and 70 percent will die of the disease. However, if the cancer is found and treated before it has spread, the five-year survival rate is 94 percent (2011). A small percent of ovarian cancer is hereditary. Gilda Radner, a *Saturday Night Live* comedian, died of misdiagnosed familial ovarian cancer, making the disease publicly recognized.

Ovarian cancer is the deadliest of all gynecologic cancers and is often referred to as the "silent killer" because the symptoms can be mistaken for many other common ailments. Symptoms of fatigue, gas, and bloating may go unrecognized. To compound the problem, no specific tests are available that screen for ovarian cancer. Many women end up seeing a gastroenterologist, who may incorrectly diagnose irritable bowel syndrome. Because of the elusive symptoms, only a small percent of all ovarian cancers are detected at an early stage. If you have symptoms that may indicate ovarian cancer, insist on a few simple blood tests—CA125 and BRCA1 or BRCA2. While these tests are not conclusive, they are a start.

When ovarian cancer symptoms are present, they are persistent and worsen with time. Symptoms of ovarian cancer often mimic those of many other common conditions, including digestive and bladder problems. They include

- abdominal pressure, fullness, swelling, or bloating;
- pelvic discomfort or pain;
- persistent indigestion, gas, or nausea;
- changes in bowel and bladder habits, including a frequent need to urinate;
- loss of appetite or quickly feeling full;

- increased abdominal girth or clothes fitting tighter around your waist;
- a persistent lack of energy; and
- low back pain.

If you are diagnosed with ovarian cancer, get a second or third opinion and find a cancer surgeon who is a specialist in ovarian cancer—a gynecological oncologist. These two websites provide helpful information and resources:

- Ovarian Cancer National Alliance (www.ovariancancer.org)
- National Ovarian Cancer Coalition (www.ovarian.org)

As with breast cancer, the staging of ovarian cancer is just as important as early detection and diagnosis. An inaccurate staging diagnosis may cause an overly aggressive treatment that could lead to additional noncancer problems or cause a terminal patient to lose quality of life. However, a treatment that is not aggressive enough could cause further spread of cancer.

Unnecessary Hysterectomies

Unnecessary hysterectomies are perhaps the most common abuse of women in the health care system. A hysterectomy is the most commonly performed nonobstetric surgery in America and experts estimate that 75 percent of these procedures are unnecessary.

According to The Hysterectomy Educational Resources and Services (HERS) Foundation's adverse effects data bank, "99.7 percent of women in an ongoing study were given little or no prior information about the acknowledged adverse effects of hysterectomy—information that is a legal requisite of consent"(2011). A hysterectomy leaves a woman unable to have children, changes hormonal levels, may affect sexuality, and may initiate early menopause. Studies find that a hysterectomy with removal of the ovaries leads to a greater risk of heart disease. Such surgeries may also result in damage to the bladder and bowels.

Misdiagnosis in Women

Many conditions share symptoms, and it can be misleading if not all the symptoms present themselves or if the symptoms come and go. This makes it easy for your doctor to make a misdiagnosis. In the following four conditions, as many as one in five diagnoses are either incorrect or go undiagnosed:

Heart Attacks

Women are just as vulnerable to heart attacks as men. Women's heart attack symptoms are different from those of men, and they are more likely to be dismissed and misdiagnosed by doctors. Physicians often interpret cardiac illness warning signs as heartburn or symptoms of anxiety disorders. Women are more likely to die from sudden cardiac death than men are, and according to the National Heart, Lung and Blood Institute, "twenty three percent die within one year after having a heart attack" (2007). Furthermore, women are also more likely to have other conditions including diabetes, high blood pressure, or high cholesterol—all of which make a misdiagnosis more probable.

Symptoms of heart attacks are not the only things that differ between men and women. Women are less likely to believe they are having a heart attack and more likely to delay emergency treatment.

What are the signs of a heart attack? Many people think a heart attack is sudden and intense, where a person grabs his or her chest and falls over. Many heart attacks start slowly as a mild pain or discomfort. If you feel such a symptom, you may not be sure what's wrong. Symptoms may even come and go.

The following are signs of a woman's impending heart attack and should not be ignored: Most women report overwhelming fatigue in the month before their heart attack yet are unable to sleep. They also report feeling extremely anxious, stressed, and keyed up, and they describe it as a feeling of "impending doom." They also experience indigestion, nausea, and stomach pain, and other digestive disruptions; feel extremely short of breath when doing regular daily tasks; suffer from clammy, sweaty skin and a light-headed or weak feeling and other sudden flulike symptoms.

While pain and numbness in the chest, shoulder, or arm is a typical sign of heart attack among men, women experience the pain more as a sensation of tightness running along their jaw and down the neck and sometimes up to the ear. The pain may extend down to the shoulder and arm, especially on the left side, or could feel similar to a bad backache or pulled muscle in the neck or back.

If you feel heart attack symptoms, do not delay. Remember, minutes matter! Do not wait for more than a few minutes to call 911. If you just don't feel right, do not be afraid to see a professional right away. You know your own body, so if you feel "off" and know that something is wrong, don't allow your doctor to overlook or brush off your symptoms. Your future health depends on your vigilance, knowledge, and early intervention.

Hormonal Imbalances

Hormonal imbalances are frequently misdiagnosed in women. For example, thyroid disease affects about one in eight women yet is often mistaken for depression. Mood swings, weight gain, and rapid heartbeat can be misattributed to lack of exercise and poor diet habits. Physicians also mistake the complaints of rapid heartbeats or moodiness in young women as being that of a heart condition or of common depression. Women who develop a hormonal imbalance at a young age and who are not diagnosed or treated are at high risk for developing severe osteoporosis later in life, chronic heart disease, and many other health risks. The only one way to know for sure if you are suffering from a hormonal imbalance is through simple blood testing.

Autoimmune Diseases

Symptoms of rheumatoid arthritis, multiple sclerosis, lupus, and fibromyalgia are common among women and are often misdiagnosed as too much stress. Fatigue and joint pain can also be signs of anxiety or depression, which many autoimmune-disease sufferers are told they have. Autoimmune diseases often follow a pattern in which the symptoms get worse and then get better, or go away completely. These periods alternate with each other and often get worse, making for an easy misdiagnosis.

Endometriosis

This illness can cause crippling cramps and eventual infertility and is frequently diagnosed as an irregular menstrual cycle. Women may be told the pain is "in their head" while others are under the wrong impression that painful periods are normal. According to *Endometriosis.org*, a recent survey found that it takes an average of eight years for a woman to get an endometriosis diagnosis. Of those women, 65 percent received a misdiagnosis of another disease, and up to 50 percent had to see five or more medical professionals before they receive an accurate diagnosis (2011).

Ways to Improve Your Risks of Receiving a Misdiagnosis

To reduce the chance of receiving a misdiagnosis, bring a trusted friend or family member with you to the doctor's office to take notes. Allow this person to ask questions you may forget or are too embarrassed to ask. The only way to get an accurate diagnosis is by sharing accurate information even though it is sometimes embarrassing to discuss sensitive symptoms.

When you arrive at a doctor's appointment with a list of symptoms and questions, your doctor will find it difficult to rush out the door with unanswered questions still on your list. If you don't understand what your doctor is saying, stop the conversation, and ask questions until you fully understand.

Without history and background knowledge, it is much harder for a stand-in doctor to understand you as a whole person. That's why it is important to see the same practitioner each time you visit the doctor.

Doctors are less likely to look for a serious diagnosis if you are young and in good health. If you don't fit the typical demographic, your illness may be overlooked. Keep this in mind if you do not fit the "normal" illness profile.

Sometimes it is difficult to avoid the parent-child relationship that is typical between doctors and patients. Approach every appointment as an adult working with another adult. Do not allow yourself to feel subservient. This is no time to be shy or demure. Do your homework and come to each doctor visit armed with knowledge and assertiveness—not aggressiveness.

Your doctor has not seen everything. Usually, doctors see about three hundred different diagnoses throughout the course of their practice. This leaves a lot of room for error. When your doctor announces your diagnosis, always ask, "What else could it be?"

If your doctor prescribes diagnostic testing, be sure to understand the procedure, the risks, and the outcomes the test can discover and do not hesitate to get a second opinion. Your health is not the time to worry about hard feelings. Any worthwhile doctor should encourage you to understand your diagnosis and your need to feel comfortable about your options.

Prescription Drugs

The drugs, Prempro, Premarin, Provera and other drugs used in hormone replacement therapy (HRT) are known to cause breast cancer. Prempro is linked to serious side effects in women including breast cancer, stroke, blood clots, and cardiovascular disease. A long-term study by the National Heart, Lung, and Blood Institute (NHLBI) that consisted of more than 16,000 women between the ages of fifty and seventy-nine discovered that women who were given Prempro were much more likely to develop serious health problems compared to women in the placebo group (2005). The study, originally planned to last eight years, ended after only five years when researchers determined the side effects of Prempro were so severe that they could no longer continue to subject the participants to the dangerous drug.

Many doctors are so busy with their practices, they have little time to understand how the potential side effects might interact negatively with you as a unique individual. Often they rely on the free samples and "marketing wisdom" of their drug reps, who have no understanding of diseases, medicine, or patient needs.

When a female patient presents herself at the doctor's office with symptoms of depression and headaches, does the doctor routinely ask about a potential pregnancy before prescribing Paxil, Zoloft, or

Topamax? The use of the drugs Paxil, Zoloft, and other antidepressants may increase a child's risk of birth defects when taken during pregnancy. In addition, the Food and Drug Administration issued a birth defects warning for Topomax, a migraine and epilepsy drug.

Similarly, the prescription painkiller Vioxx was recalled after a clinical trial indicated that those taking the drug had double the risk of a heart attack, stroke, or sudden death as those taking a placebo. How many patients have died because of "free" samples of Vioxx promoted by the solicitation of a drug rep?

Part of the prescription drug problem is because pharmacies can legally sell doctors' prescribing information to data miners and drug companies. The American Medical Association (AMA) also sells their data, called the prescription master file, and in doing so, makes millions of dollars each year in royalties. The data miners buy all the prescription records from the pharmacies, and the AMA master file. The data miners combine this information and sell it to drug companies. That's how the sales rep knows that Dr. ABC wrote ten prescriptions on Friday, what brand they were, and what drugstore filled them.

According to a recent online post from the *New England Journal of Medicine*,

> Being able to identify prescribing patterns is very powerful to the companies. If they send in a drug detailer with a certain tactic, or if they meet with the doctor at a convention, or if they hire the doctor to give speeches, the company can track in real time, every day, the impact of all these activities. If a certain doctor is given free samples of a drug, they can then track over the next weeks or months whether the doctor has written new prescriptions for the drug. If the doctor doesn't, they can go in and try to modify their behavior. They can 'punish' doctors who are not writing the scripts and reward those who do. If they know a doctor has recently switched and is prescribing more of a rival drug, they can go in and say something negative about the rival drug. Data mining raises questions as to whether physicians are being inappropriately influenced. That's why medical societies and journals are concerned. They want to protect the integrity

of the physician's prescription process. They want doctors to be making decisions based on the clinical facts, with their patient, not based on the fact that the drug company knows too much about them. (2011)

Because of these tactics, you should be curious about suspicious alliances. If your doctor gives you free samples, ask about other similar drugs. Ask why he or she prescribes this particular one. Before you take any drug, research it online, study the side effects, and question your doctor and your pharmacist about other alternatives. Sometimes you may have no other choice but to take a certain drug to cure an illness. Use good judgment, and do not take prescribed medication without understanding all of the potential implications, just because your doctor says so.

Pregnancy and Birthing

Birth injuries to both mother and infant can occur because doctors are trained to intervene in an effort to relieve birth pain or to hurry a birth along to fit hospital scheduling. Staff shortages, incorrect treatment, and the overuse of pain-relieving drugs contribute to birth complications. It is important to know how doctor intervention during pregnancy and labor can result in negative outcomes:

- Misdiagnosis of gestational diabetes or high blood pressure—pre-eclampsia
- Failure to diagnose and treat pulmonary edema in women with pre-eclampsia
- Failure to control blood pressure in hypertensive women
- Failure to recognize pre-existing medical conditions
- Miscalculation of contractions
- Improper administration of Pitocin and other labor inducing drugs, causing a ruptured uterus
- Giving the wrong drugs
- Improper epidural that weakens contractions and carries the risk of paralysis

- Failure to order a C-section in time to avoid high-risk complications
- Failure to take or pay attention to vital signs, especially following a C-section
- Hemorrhage following C-section
- Lack of measures for the prevention of venous thromboembolism before C-section

Have a written birth plan that includes acceptable emergency intervention methods that both you and your doctor agree upon ahead of time. This can alleviate many problems.

Prevent a Hospital Stay

There are many ways to stay out of the hospital. The time to think about prevention and wellness is sooner rather than later. Linda Garvin RN, MSN, a nurse patient advocate and the owner of Patient Advocate Bay Area, Inc., in Alameda, California, says, "Wellness issues can be a constant worry—from not getting enough sleep, to problem ingredients in cosmetics, to choosing healthy foods or to not getting the right kinds of exercise. An experienced health advocate can help you explore treatment options and develop wellness strategies."

Your health is especially fragile after a hospital stay, a surgery, or an illness. Linda shares a story she received from a former client named Shelly. Shelly says, "I was diagnosed with breast cancer that required radiation therapy along with a lumpectomy. I felt that I needed the expertise of a nurse to get some questions answered and to help me review my treatment options, so I contacted Linda. Prior to surgery, Linda helped me prepare for my physician appointments with specific and focused questions. She supplied several reading resources on breast cancer—easy to access and understand. She also helped me to find treatment options. After surgery and radiation, I needed further help to make lifestyle changes that could lower my risk for additional health problems. Linda provided me with information about proper diets choices, cooking methods to decrease inflammation and food shopping tips. Because of her guidance and coaching, I now understand how to choose safer personal care products and manage my physical and emotional stress by incorporating regular exercise and mind-body techniques. Now I manage my health in ways I didn't think were possible thanks to Linda's compassionate support and straightforward proactive health strategies.

In addition to wellness coaching, screening tests are valuable tools that look for diseases before you have symptoms. Here are some essential screening tests—however if you have other concerning symptoms or conditions, get regular screenings for those too:

Breast Cancer

Ask your doctor if a mammogram is right for you based on your age, family history, health, and other personal concerns.

Cervical Cancer

Have a Pap smear on a regular basis as suggested by your doctor.

Chlamydia and Other Sexually Transmitted Diseases

Have a screening test for chlamydia if you are twenty-four or younger and sexually active. If you are older than twenty-four years old, talk to your doctor about the need for a chlamydia and other sexually transmitted disease screenings.

Colorectal Cancer

Have a screening test for colorectal cancer starting at age fifty. If you have a family history of colorectal cancer, you may need to be screened earlier.

Diabetes

Get screened for diabetes if your blood pressure is higher than 135/80 or if you take medication for high blood pressure.

Depression

Mental health is often overlooked. Depression can be caused by a variety of reasons including stress, biological and hormonal causes, body image issues, psychological reasons, and others. If you feel sad, anxious, apathetic, sleep or eat more than usual or exhibit other signs of depression, see your doctor. Hypothyroidism, an under-active thyroid, can cause depression, so rule this out if you are feeling depressed.

High Blood Pressure

Have your blood pressure checked on a regular basis as suggested by your doctor. High blood pressure can cause stroke, heart attack, kidney and eye problems, and heart failure.

High Cholesterol

Have your cholesterol checked regularly if you use tobacco, you are obese, you have diabetes or high blood pressure, you have a personal history of heart disease or blocked arteries, or as suggested by your doctor.

HIV

Talk with your doctor about HIV screening if you have any risk or lifestyle factors.

Osteoporosis (Bone Thinning)

If you are younger than sixty-five years old, talk to your doctor about your testing needs.

Overweight and Obesity

If you are obese, find ways to change your behaviors to help lose weight in a safe and healthy manner.

Preventive care is the best way to avoid a hospital stay. However, because of multiple sources of responsibilities and stresses, many women put off their own health care to care for others. Studies reveal that women are most often caregivers to ill or older family members and are usually the decision maker when it comes to children or spouse's health care. Add to that, women's health care can be disjointed because of multiple providers—OB-GYN for women's health issues and a primary care physician for others. All of these reasons and more can compete with attaining quality personal health care. Women can do much to prevent illness by being aware of the unique pitfalls that surround their health and by taking the time to take care.

CHAPTER 10

Children's Challenges

HEALTH care for children is not as safe as it should or could be. There is very little information about hospital safety issues in children's health care because the majority of their health care takes place in nonhospital settings—pediatrician's offices, emergency departments, outpatient settings, and at home. Additionally, children receive care from a variety of providers, including daycare, schools, parents, and others. In these settings, health care safety may not even exist.

Children rely on their care from the adults in their life who may conflict—parents, stepparents, guardians, relatives, school administrators, or babysitters. Because of the diversity and informality of these settings and providers, children's health care safety is especially susceptible to errors in handoffs. A handoff occurs anytime care is transferred from one person to another or from one location to another, and handoffs are ripe for miscommunication.

The hospital setting presents additional challenges, due to multiple environments and transfer opportunities—from the emergency department to the pediatric intensive care unit or from childbirth to neonatal intensive care. During these handoff times, the coordination of care is paramount.

A study titled *Medication Errors and Adverse Drug Events in Pediatric Inpatients* assessed the rates of pediatric medication errors, adverse drug events, and potential adverse drug events. Seven hundred and seventy eight medication orders were reviewed. The study showed 616 medical errors, 115 potential adverse drug events, and twenty-six actual adverse drug events. Shockingly, the potential adverse drug rate was three times higher in children than in adults. Most of the problems occurred at the point of drug ordering and dispensing and involved incorrect dosing (79 percent) due to ordering high or low doses of medication. Ordering medications despite known allergies and without indicating the route of administration were other serious mistakes, as well as incorrect dispensing of pharmacy medications, with intravenous fluids as the biggest culprit (54 percent). The main cause of error was human error because of heavy workload, distractions, and inexperienced staff. The study's conclusion states, "Medication errors are common in pediatric inpatient settings, and further efforts are needed to reduce them" (2001).

Because infants and children are such high-risk patients, the need for a round-the-clock advocate is profound. Given that medication errors top the list—parents, family, and advocates must understand all aspects of potential adverse drug events. Make the hospital staff aware of any medications or treatments your child is taking at home. Know the dosage and what the pills, liquids, and IVs look like. Make sure the medications are taken as prescribed and on time. Know what drugs to continue at home, how to administer them, and for how long.

Beware of antibiotic misuse and overuse. In the article, *The relationship between perceived parental expectations and pediatrician antimicrobial prescribing behavior*, published by the American Academy of Pediatrics, a pediatric study showed that doctors prescribe antibiotics 62 percent of the time if they perceive parents expect them and only 7 percent of the time if they feel parents do not expect them (1999). Antibiotics fight bacterial infections. Antibiotics do not fight infections caused by viruses, namely the common cold, flu, most coughs, bronchitis or sore throat, unless a culture indicates a strep infection.

Birth Injuries

Birth injuries often occur when the infant is deprived of oxygen, causing brain damage. If the doctor does not promptly deliver a baby in distress, or if a baby is not resuscitated moments after birth, there is a possibility that the resulting lack of oxygen will cause serious brain damage. Another dangerous risk involves the improper use of equipment. X-ray and imaging devices should be set to lower levels of radiation, and all equipment thoroughly sanitized to avoid the spread of disease or infection. Other common birth injuries are:

- *Cerebral palsy*—a disorder caused by trauma to the brain during or near the time of birth. The damage done to the brain determines the severity. A variety of medical mistakes including the improper use of forceps or leaving the baby in the birth canal for too long can cause cerebral palsy.
- *Shoulder dystocia*—misdiagnosis or delayed diagnosis of gestational diabetes can increase the risk of shoulder dystocia, a situation where the baby's head is delivered and the shoulders become trapped under the mother's pelvic floor.
- *Erb's palsy/brachial plexus injuries*—a paralysis or weakness of the arm caused by stretching of the nerves around the shoulder during birth. This damage can be caused by excessive pulling on the arm during birth or by pressure on the baby's raised shoulders during a breech delivery.

Your obstetrician plays an important part in the delivery of your baby. It is crucial for him or her to communicate with you about any possible complications. Have an advocate in the birthing room with you at all times to watch for potential problems you may otherwise miss during such a heavily charged emotional and physical time.

Tips to Prevent Medical Care Errors in Children

The Joint Commission has a brochure that highlights how to prevent errors in your child's care. They make the following excellent suggestions.

To prepare for your child's visit to the doctor's office or hospital, it is helpful to make a written list of your child's medical history. Include vaccinations, allergies, current health problems, and the dates of any surgeries and hospital visits. Make another list of your child's medicines. Include prescription and over-the-counter medicines, vitamins, and herbs. Be sure to include the amount your child takes. Include general and specific questions you have about your child's health.

When consulting with your doctor, find out about all the tests and treatments for your child's illness or injury. Ask how a treatment works and understand that more tests or treatments are not always better. If you do not fully understand what your doctor is saying, tell the doctor you do not understand. Tell the doctor if you need someone who speaks your language.

To prevent your child from getting an infection, remind caregivers to wash or clean their hands before touching your child. Hand washing helps prevent infection. Remind caregivers to wear clean gloves when they draw blood, touch wounds, or examine your child's body.

To prevent errors in your child's care, use medicines safely. Tell the doctor or nurse your child's current weight or ask them to weigh your child (in kilograms). Medicines for children are based on weight.

Ask the following questions:

- Why does my child need a new medicine? How will it help?
- What are the names of the medicine?
- Is there written information about the medicine?
- What does the medicine look like? Is it a liquid or a pill? What color is the medicine?
- How do I give my child this medicine? (You should be able to repeat the instructions back to the caregiver.)
- Can I cut or crush pills or put them in food if my child has trouble swallowing them? (Certain medicines may not work or may be harmful if cut or crushed. Ask if the medicine comes in a liquid or can be given another way.)
- What are the side effects?

Remind the doctor or caregiver about your child's allergies and reactions to any medicines in the past. Tell the doctor or caregiver if you do not understand any information or if you have questions. When you get the medicine, check the label for your child's name, the correct medicine name, dosage and directions.

If your child has a medical tests, X-ray, MRI, CT scan, or laboratory test (including a blood or urine test), ask why your child needs it. Get information about the test and preparation instructions. Find out if you can be with your child during the test. Ask if your child can eat or drink before the test. If your child is having an X-ray, MRI, or CT scan, ask if your child will be given a contrast agent. This liquid makes organs and blood vessels easy to see on X-rays and other tests. Tell the staff if your child has had problems with contrast agents before. Immediately alert staff if your child begins to itch or have trouble breathing after getting a contrast agent.

Ask about any risks associated with the medical or lab tests. X-rays and CT scans use radiation, so ask how they will make sure your child gets the right amount of radiation for his or her size. MRIs use strong magnets. Metal can be pulled into the MRI machine and injure the patient. Make sure to remove all metal-like jewelry, hair clips, or toys with metal parts. If you are unsure, ask the staff. Also ask about safety protocols to make sure your child is safe during the test.

If your child is having a blood test, urine test, or other lab test, ask to see the label on the container. The label should have your child's name and birth date or another piece of information. See that the container is immediately sealed.

To help prevent errors in the hospital, check your child's identification band. Make sure the information on the band is correct. Make sure caregivers check the band and ask your child's name before giving any medicine, test, or treatment. Caregivers should also ask for your child's birth date or other identifying information.

If your child is staying overnight at the hospital, insist on staying too. Most hospitals will let a parent stay overnight. It is important that you or someone you trust be with your child whenever possible to be their advocate.

If your child needs an IV, remember that an IV should not be left in any longer than needed to avoid infection. Ask to have the IV removed as soon as possible. Tell caregivers if the IV area is painful, red, or puffy.

Here are additional tips to help you and your child during a hospital stay: All staff should wear an identification badge. Ask to see a badge if you cannot see it. If your child is in pain, tell the staff immediately; they should check your child regularly for pain. If your child moves to another floor or department, check that your child gets the correct medicines and treatments after the move. Alert caregivers if you think there is any confusion. Ask visitors who are ill to call on the phone or come back when they are well.

If your child is having surgery, talk to the surgeon and others who will be in the operating room. It is important that you are confident in the ability of the people who will operate on your child. Before an operation, ask the surgeon to mark the body part while you are in the room. Make sure the surgeon marks only the correct part and nowhere else. If your child needs anesthesia for a procedure, request a pediatric anesthesiologist. Ask if you can stay with your child until the sedatives (sleep medicines) begin to work and your child falls asleep.

After the operation, ask if pediatric specialists will be caring for your child in the recovery area. Before hospital discharge, ask about the care your child will need at home. Get written instructions. Write down the names and phone numbers of people to call if you have questions or in case of an emergency (2011).

Additional Safety Tips for Newborns and Infants

Infant abductions do occur. Statistics show that most abductions take place directly from the mother's hospital room and not from the nursery. The National Center for Missing and Exploited Children released a list of all newborn and infant abductions from 1983 to 2010 made by non-family members from U.S. hospitals, homes or other areas. Of the 271 reported cases of infant abductions, a whopping forty seven percent of the incidents occurred in hospital facilities. The majority of those infants (58 percent) were taken from their mother's hospital room.

According to a paper, "Guidelines on Prevention of and Response to Infant Abductions" by John B. Rabun of the National Center for Missing & Exploited Children,

> The typical abduction from a health care facility involves an "unknown" abductor impersonating a nurse, health care employee, volunteer, or relative in order to gain access to an infant. The obstetrics unit is an open and inviting one where patients' decreased length of stay, from one to three days, gives them less time to know staff members. In addition, it can be filled with medical and nursing staff members, visitors, students, volunteers, and participants in parenting and newborn-care classes. The number of new and changing faces on the unit is

high, thus making the unit an area where a "stranger" is unlikely to be noticed. Because there is generally easier access to a mother's room than to the newborn nursery and a newborn infant spends increasingly more time with his or her mother rather than in the traditional nursery setting, most abductors "con" the infant directly from the mother's arms. (2009)

The following are additional tips to keep you and your baby safe from a hospital "code pink" announcement:

- Make sure the hospital takes protective measures to identify your baby; these include footprinting, color photos or videos, or sample of your infant's cord blood.
- Do not give your baby to anyone who does not have a hospital photo ID badge.
- Check every badge to see if the staff member's face matches the face on the ID before you hand over your child. When a staff member brings your baby to you, verify that the name and information on the baby's band is correct.
- Do not carry your baby in the hallways. Use the approved bassinet.
- When a staff member comes to take your baby, ask where the child is going and why. Get every detail about the intended test or procedure and accompany your child as far as you can. Ask if you can be present during the procedures. If not, stay by the door to watch for who comes in and who goes out.
- When the baby is in your room, remain in the room with the baby. Do not leave the child unattended or with family members except a spouse or someone you trust.
- If you use the bathroom while your baby is in the room, keep the door open enough to see the crib. If you must sleep while your baby is in the room, keep the crib next to your bed on the opposite side of the door. Hang a bell or other noisemaking object on the crib so that if someone moves it, you will wake up.

Children are not little adults. They have distinct needs and require special attention because of their inexperience and inability to advocate for themselves. During a hospital stay, it becomes especially important to have an adult advocate present at all times.

CHAPTER 11

Vigilance for Veterans

THIS chapter is born out of my personal experience as I watched an aging family member, Louise, care for her veteran husband, Harold. Harold suffered from posttraumatic stress disorder caused by his time spent in the Navy during World War II and eventually he developed Alzheimer's disease. Louise was his caretaker and did everything she could to protect his dignity. No one in the family was aware of his frequent "nightmares" or knew that he couldn't order off the menu at a restaurant without assistance. When Harold said something that was incongruous to the conversation, Louise would laugh and say, "Oh, Harold!" as if he was just trying to be funny. Louise's job was to keep him safe.

On one of our Navy reunion trips, Louise didn't seem to be herself, yet she quietly kept her focus and attention on Harold. Six months later, she was diagnosed with terminal leukemia. Only when close to dying did she reveal she had experienced symptoms before the reunion trip. She felt that if she took the time to care for herself, who would look after Harold?

As I was planning the chapters for this book, her story came to mind. I wondered if she would be alive today if she heeded the early warning signs and taken the time to care for herself. With over 20 million veterans in the United States today, how many other caregivers experience the same thing? My goal for this chapter is to show the differences between caregivers of veterans and caregivers of nonveterans and to give both veterans and their caregivers tools to keep them safe and out of a hospital.

According to the report of findings taken from the Caregivers of
Veterans—Serving on the Home Front study,

> The distinct nature of a Veteran's illness or injury drives different
> caregiving needs than those of non-Veteran caregivers. In addi-
> tion, there is a huge disparity in caregiver demographics. Ninety
> six percent of caregivers of Veterans are women compared to
> the national number of 65 percent woman. Seventy percent of
> Veteran caregivers provide care to their spouse or partner versus
> the national figure of only 6 percent who provide care to their
> spouse or partner. Some of the newly injured are in their twenties,
> with caregivers who may be parents entering their 50s and 60s
> and face decades in this role. The youngest Veterans requiring
> caregivers, those whose ranks are growing from Operation Iraqi
> Freedom and Operation Enduring Freedom in Afghanistan,
> pose a particular concern. One in four is being cared for by their
> parents. As their parents age, they will likely need more care-
> giving support and, ultimately, caregiving responsibilities may
> need to be transitioned to others.

> The medical conditions for which Veterans need care differ
> greatly from the typical population too. The types of health
> conditions from which the Veteran is suffering vary in close rela-
> tion to the Veteran's age and the war in which he or she served.
> Caregivers of older Veterans and those serving in Vietnam or
> earlier increasingly report the presence of diabetes or cancer.
> Both conditions are more common among Veterans than in a
> similarly aged general population. A large proportion of Veterans
> have mental illness such as depression or anxiety (70%) or post
> traumatic stress disorder (PTSD) (60%), whereas nationally,
> mental or emotional health problems are reported by only 28
> percent. Depression/anxiety, PTSD and spinal cord injuries are
> more common among younger Veterans, particularly those who
> served in Vietnam or later. Other conditions include traumatic
> brain injury (TBI), diabetes, and paralysis, loss of limb or spinal
> cord injury. Of note, eight in ten caregivers report their Veteran

has two or more specific conditions and two-thirds name additional conditions such as bone, joint, or limb problems, hearing or ear problems, heart conditions, and neuropathy/nerve issues. Thus, strategies to inform, educate, and support caregivers must address multiple needs. Care for a Veteran whose condition is service-related is a longer-term endeavor than family caregiving typically is, with 30 percent of caregivers of Veterans having been in their role for 10 years or more, compared to only 15 percent nationally.

Not only are caregivers of Veterans in their role for a longer period, but their burden of care is also heavier. Sixty five percent are in a high burden caregiving situation compared to 31 percent nationally. The increased burden is due to a greater likelihood of helping with Activities of Daily Living including dressing, bathing, feeding, and incontinence as well as housework, managing finances, transportation, grocery shopping, preparing meals and giving medications.

In addition caregivers help the Veterans with other aspects of their care and with day-to-day living. Nearly all of those who care for a Veteran with TBI, PTSD, or depression/ anxiety say they help him or her cope with stressful situations or avoid "triggers" of anxiety or anti-social behavior. Nearly nine out of ten of all caregivers of Veterans say they advocate for him/her with care providers, government agencies, or schools, remind or give cues about what he/she should be doing and coordinate medical care and rehabilitative services. A considerable share administers physical or medical therapies and treatments.

Perhaps because of their increased burden of care, caregivers of Veterans report a greater impact of caregiving on their lives than caregivers in general do. Moreover, the caregivers of Veterans who have PTSD, TBI, or mental illness such as depression or anxiety are even more likely to suffer many impacts of caregiving—on health, emotional stress, feelings of isolation, the caregiver's marriage and children, and finances. The heightened impact of providing care to a Veteran is manifest in a number of ways. Overall, twice as many caregivers of Veterans consider their caregiving situation to be highly stressful than do caregivers of adults nationwide (68% vs. 31%) and three times as many say there is a high degree of physical strain (40% vs. 14%). Of those who are currently married, separated, or divorced, three-quarters say caregiving or the Veteran's condition placed a strain on their marriage. Among the 30 percent who have children under the age of 18 in the household, two-thirds report having spent less time with their children than they would like and 57 percent report that their children or grandchildren had emotional or school problems as a result of their caregiving or the Veteran's condition.

It is understandable then that providing care to a Veteran with a service-related condition has widespread impacts on the caregiver's health. Large proportions report increased stress or anxiety (88%) or sleep deprivation (77%). Caregiving activities take time that caregivers would otherwise use to take care of themselves. Healthy behaviors such as exercising, eating habits and going to one's own doctor and dentist appointments on schedule decline for roughly six in ten, and similar proportions have weight gain/loss or experience depression. Preventive health care also suffers for many, in that two-thirds spend less time exercising, 58 percent delay or skip their own doctor or dentist appointments and more than half lapse into poor eating habits. Perhaps as a result of these behavioral changes, 66 percent gain or lose weight and 63 percent suffer from depression and generally get sick more often. (2011)

It is easy to see that caregivers of veterans may have a higher chance of hospitalization to treat their own health issues. These findings show that both veterans and their caregivers and family members face unique health care challenges and must be extra vigilant to prevent a hospital stay. The main health challenges a caregiver faces are many, including;

not knowing what to expect medically with the veteran's condition or how to treat it; not understanding how providing such constant high-touch care can affect his or her own personal health; and lastly, not knowing where to turn for specialized care or to arrange for a break from caregiving.

Ways to Help Your Veteran

Caregivers play an important part in keeping their veterans out of the hospital. If you are a caregiver, make sure you are in the loop when health decisions are made. Know what you are up against and learn about the disease, condition, or injury affecting the veteran you care for.

Talk to the veteran's health care provider, and ask the following questions: Is this a long-term or short-term situation? What are the veteran's care needs? Will those needs change?

Learn about special skills that you may need to care for your veteran. Your community is an excellent source for information. Talk with your local medical center staff about their services, and reach out to the county health department to inquire about available public resources. Explore options—adult day health care, meal delivery, transportation services, respite services, and in-home support services. Call your local area agency on aging and contact organizations specific to the disease. Keep the information you collect in a notebook or on the computer. Even if you don't use the information now, you may need it in the future.

Talk to your local VA Caregiver Support coordinator about resources that can help you learn more about caregiving. To find your local VA Caregiver Support coordinator, visit the "Help Near Home" page on the VA Caregiver Support website (http://www.caregiver.va.gov). Get to know the VA social worker or nurse who specializes in arranging for care. Make sure the veteran you care for is involved. Ask what he or she thinks when it comes to immediate care.

It is also important to keep track of the veteran's health and care needs. Create a log or journal of eating patterns, medications, and physical symptoms. At the very least, write down the following information and keep it nearby should an emergency arise: doctors' names, phone numbers, and addresses; medical name of the illness or injury; prescription numbers, names and doses; and pharmacy contact information.

Organize financial information, household bills, bank accounts, and insurance policies. Photocopy important information including the veteran's VA ID card, social security card, driver's license, and insurance cards. Keep these important documents where you can locate them quickly. Plan ahead by asking an attorney or your VA social worker for information on advance directives and a durable power of attorney for health care. Should a hospital stay pop up without warning, you need to have all of these important documents on hand.

If the veteran you care for must go to the hospital, arrange to have an advocate there at all times to keep him or her safe.

Ways to Keep the Caregiver out of the Hospital

If you are a caregiver, you need to stay in good health. You will not do service to your veteran if you land in the hospital. Get regular health and dental checkups and any annual health screenings you may need. Try to maintain regular sleeping patterns. Eat healthy meals and snacks. Daily physical activity can help lower stress and increase your energy. Remember, the healthier you are, the better care you will provide.

Your mental health is important, too. Connect with other caregivers who may be going through the same thing. Be realistic about what you can and cannot do. Get other family members involved to provide support. You don't have to do it all alone, and you shouldn't feel as if you have to.

If you are balancing work and caregiving, talk to your employer about flexibility in your job. You may be able to take time off from work under the Family and Medical Leave Act. This federal law allows qualified employees to take up to twelve weeks of unpaid time off to care for a family member. Talk with your employer about an Employee Assistance Program that provides support for caregivers. Find out if your employer offers flextime or work-from-home opportunities.

All caregivers feel overwhelmed at times. If you feel angry or often lose patience with the veteran you care for, ask for assistance. Seek help if you use alcohol, drugs, or medication to cope. If you are depressed, talk to a doctor, counselor, or therapist. Depression can be treated.

Caring for an ill, injured, or disabled veteran can be stressful, but it can also be incredibly rewarding. Caregiving offers you a chance to give back to someone important in your life.

About My HealtheVet

My HealtheVet is the VA's e-health website, which offers veterans, active duty soldiers, their dependents, and caregivers free access to VA health care information and services. With My HealtheVet, veterans can access current health and benefits information and record and store important health and military history information at their convenience.

Veterans who receive care at a VA facility should ask about In-Person Authentication (IPA). Registered users who are VA patients and have completed the IPA process can view the names of their VA prescriptions online, access their personal VA wellness reminders, view VA lab results and communicate with their providers through secure messaging. For more information, visit My HealtheVet at www.myhealth.va.gov.

To find a family caregiver support group, call the VA Caregiver Support Line (1-855-260-3247), your local faith establishment, or other local groups to learn about support groups in your area.

CHAPTER 12

Holistic Healing

HOLISTIC healing is a state of mind and a lifestyle. It's about looking at yourself as a "whole" person—physically, mentally, emotionally and spiritually. When you are in tune with yourself, you can listen to your body to detect when it becomes off balance. Complementary and alternative medicine (CAM) allows you to take charge of your health and influence your health outcomes. You have control over how you choose to perceive and react to any situation and have the ability to choose your thoughts to influence your body's responses.

The mind cannot distinguish between what is real and what is not. For example, it cannot tell the difference between the happy and carefree feeling you have when you are physically on the beach versus the thought or memory of being on the beach. This connection can accomplish amazing results. The time to think about this is right now. Don't wait for a looming illness or hospital stay. Begin today to choose how you perceive your everyday situations and stresses. If you are the patient or the advocate, take advantage of your ability to remain in control and stay healthy.

Many people use complementary and alternative medicine in pursuit of health and well-being. The National Center for Complementary and Alternative Health describes CAM as a group of diverse medical and health care practices, systems, and products that are not generally considered part of regular medicine. *Complementary medicine* refers to practices used "in tandem" **with** conventional medicine, such as using acupuncture in addition to usual care to help lessen pain. *Alternative medicine* is a practice used **"in place" of** conventional medicine. *Integrative medicine* is a practice that combines or integrates conventional with complementary and alternative treatments.

CAM practices are often grouped into broad categories—mind-body medicine, manipulative and body-based practices, and natural products. Although these categories are not formally defined, they are helpful when discussing CAM practices. CAM practices may fit into more than one category. While I am not suggesting alternative techniques as a replacement for traditional medical care—they are powerful, inexpensive, and safe ways to participate in your own health care in a positive way. The best way to decide which methods work best for you is to try them.

Mind-Body Medicine

Mind-body practices focus on the intent to use the mind to affect physical functioning and promote health. Many CAM practices embody this concept in different ways. Examples of mind-body techniques are meditation, guided imagery, positive affirmations, yoga, and tai chi, among others.

Meditation

Meditation techniques include postures, focused attention, or an open attitude toward distractions. Studies show that meditation can lower stress hormones, blood pressure, and heart rate while improving blood circulation. People use meditation to increase calmness and relaxation, improve psychological balance, cope with illness, or enhance overall health and well-being. For patient advocates, meditation can be your friend. Many times during my mom's hospital stay, I took a few minutes to go outside in the beautiful courtyard. I sat and watched the birds and meditated in my own way. These moments were refreshing and allowed me to go back inside to face the unknown.

Mindful Breathing

Breathing has a powerful influence over your physiological and psychological well-being. The way you breathe has a powerful effect on how stressed you feel. When you are under stress, your breathing tends to become rapid and shallow, and it comes from your upper chest.

Relaxed abdominal breathing, on the other hand, is a slow, calm style of breathing that originates from your diaphragm and abdomen area, with very little chest movement.

Studies show that practicing this style of abdominal breathing reduces muscle tension and anxiety in less than one minute. Breathing affects your nervous and digestive systems, your heart, muscles, sleep, energy levels, concentration, and memory. When you breathe slowly and deeply, you bring air down into the lower portion of the lungs, where the oxygen exchange is most efficient. This causes your heart rate and blood pressure to decrease. Studies also link focused breathing with reduced hot flashes in menopausal women, relief from chronic pain and headache pain, and reduced symptoms of PMS. Mindful abdominal breathing after surgery is imperative to improve lung function to avoid pneumonia.

Here is a quick way to see how you normally breathe. Imagine for a moment that you are at your doctor's office. He or she has a stethoscope and tells you, "Take a deep breath." Did you just expand your chest and raise your shoulders as you loudly inhaled?

Here is another way to test your breathing. Place one hand on your chest and place the other hand on your abdomen. Breathe normally and notice which hand is moving most. If the hand on your abdomen is moving and the hand on your upper chest is still, you are using your diaphragm. That's good. If your upper chest hand is moving more than the hand on your abdomen, then you are breathing with your chest, and this is a form of stressful breathing.

To take an abdominal breath; sit or stand in a comfortable position with your back straight and your feet flat on the floor; inhale slowly through your nose, counting to six; and exhale slowly through the mouth, counting to eight.

If you're not sure you're doing it right, put your hand on your abdomen and check to feel if it moves with every inhale and exhale. When exhaling, give a slightly audible sigh to give you an extra feeling of letting go. Remember to exhale a little longer than your inhale and to breathe rhythmically instead of deeply.

Many other breathing exercises and variations use abdominal breathing. One of them is pursed lip breathing. This is similar to the exercise above. This time, as you exhale, purse your lips as if you are going to whistle and then exhale very slowly through your pursed lips. You should push the breath out slowly about two or three times longer than your inhale.

When you modify your breathing by taking slow, deep abdominal breaths, you have the ability to control your nervous system, ease stress, alleviate hypertension symptoms, and generally feel better. I recently tested this for myself. I was having some scary digestive and throat symptoms that warranted an exploratory endoscopy. My appointment was at 7:30 AM; the doctor did not arrive until close to 8:00 AM. I was prepped, ready for the anesthesia, and left alone to wait in the procedure room. Hooked to the blood pressure and pulse machine, I watched the display screen above me. As each minute on the giant wall clock ticked by, my blood pressure numbers climbed.

I decided to practice tai chi movements in my mind. I concentrated on deep abdominal breathing. Sure enough, my blood pressure and pulse rate fell into my normal range. Just for fun, I deliberately stopped breathing properly and altered my thoughts. I looked at the long tube sitting next to me, waiting to go down my throat and scanned the room for other intimidating tools. Sure enough, my pulse rate jumped and my blood pressure increased. This was not a scientific study, yet it proved I did have control of my body's physical reactions.

Guided Imagery

Research shows that guided imagery and relaxation can decrease anxiety and pain and possibly shorten your hospital stay. Guided imagery is often presented on an audio recording or CD program in which you are guided to use your imagination to induce peace, calm, strength, and control. Using calming music, positive verbal suggestions, and relaxation cues aimed to release tension from specific parts of the body, you follow along and let the images of your mind guide you to a calm and relaxing place.

During a hospital stay, both the patient and the advocate experience fear, panic, stress, and uncertainty. Guided imagery helps reduce these negative effects. Over two hundred research studies have explored how mind-body techniques help prepare people for surgical and medical procedures and help them to recover faster. These studies show that guided imagery may reduce stress and anxiety in patients before and after surgical and medical procedures.

Many hospitals either supply or allow you to bring your own relaxation or guided imagery tools to be used before, during, and after surgery. Listen to the guided imagery program as soon as possible before your procedure, and ask your doctor if you will be able to use headphones to play your guided imagery program during your procedure. Listen to the program after your procedure, especially right after and several times each day during your recovery.

This is an important job for the patient advocate. Patient advocates should make sure the CD's are handy and explain the reasons to the nursing staff so they understand their importance. Patients should continue to listen to the program after they are discharged from the hospital for the sake of personal relaxation or to aid sleep.

Family members and patient advocates also benefit from having their own set of CDs. The patient can have his or her own program title, specific to the illness or just for healing or health in general. The advocate can use CD's that relate to stress, energy, and health. While sitting at the bedside with the patient, use headphones to relax, recharge, and reprogram your mind using guided imagery. As an advocate, you need to do all you can to take care of yourself—physically, mentally, and emotionally too.

Positive Affirmations

Positive affirmations are statements used to counteract negative thoughts and emotions. The repetition of affirmations can physically change the neural connections in your mind. They should be a part of your daily self-talk and used especially before, during, and after any surgery or medical procedure. You can buy many audio positive affirmations specific to a particular disease or problem. Or you can print your own affirmations and bring them with you to post around your hospital room. Short of that, you can simply come up with a few that are meaningful to you and repeat them to yourself throughout the day. Remember to phrase your statements as if they are true at the moment. Write and say them in the present tense. Here are a few to get you started, and they can be adapted and used by both the patient and the advocate:

- I am healthy in every way.
- I am in control of my health and wellness.
- I have abundant energy, vitality, and well-being.
- My mind is at peace.
- My body is healthy, energized, and perfect in every way.
- I am healthy and full of energy.
- I am in control of my health and wellness.

Positive affirmations are not only statements to repeat to yourself. Positive words should be used by everyone who has anything to do with you. Many times doctors and nurses stopped by Mom's room to render negative opinions about her prognosis. There was one young woman in particular who was a renal intern. She was not part of Mom's care team yet arbitrarily showed up at the foot of the bed, announcing in a loud voice, "She needs dialysis!"

These out-of-the-blue announcements alarmed my mom to the point of despair. At our next family meeting, I asked all staff to refrain from negative outbursts. Of course, it's not a good idea to hide reality from the patient; however, there is a way to speak with a positive spirit. If you are the advocate, ask your doctors and nurses to refrain from harmful comments in front of your patient. Ask to speak in the hallway and avoid hushed whispering in front of the patient. Just because the patient is asleep, appears to be asleep, is sedated, or in a coma—the subconscious mind is active and listening. Words reach the mind and have the ability to change the way the body responds.

Subliminal Programming Music

Subliminal success recordings contain positive messages or affirmations embedded in relaxing music, acted on by your mind below the level of conscious awareness. The only thing you hear is peaceful music or the calming sound of ocean waves, while underneath, thousands of positive messages are received by your subconscious mind. All you do is play the music as you go about your daily activities. Often, the CD or recording will have a "part two" that forgoes the music and subliminal suggestions. This section audibly recites the actual affirmations so you know exactly what messages your subconscious mind hears during the subliminal section.

Just the audible side of the program is enough to feed your mind positive thoughts. You do not have to accept the idea of subliminal reprogramming; however, it is commonly known that you can change your life by changing your thoughts. Subliminal programming is just one of many tools you can use to help with these changes.

When my girls were young, I played a "radiant health and a strong immune system" subliminal tape every night before bedtime. It came to be an important part of the evening routine. They seldom caught the flus or viruses that ran rampant among their friends. In fact, they went years at a time without a cold or infection. One Mother's Day, I gave my mom a copy of the same tape, and she grew to love it as much as we did. She played both the audible and subliminal sides every day as she prepared to go to work. It was only natural for me to bring the tape to the intensive care unit.

Every day I played the music repeatedly while she laid immobilized and hooked to life support. Family members of other patients gathered to inquire about the beautiful music. No one knew of subliminal programming. The nurses and hospital staff were excited and eager to make sure the tape was always playing. Each morning as I walked into the intensive care unit, the radiant health music welcomed me as it wafted down and around the hallways. That always made me smile, as I knew that not only did I believe—so did Mom's caretakers. Believing is a beautiful thing.

In addition to creating a positive mental atmosphere, the use of audio tapes and CD's can mask other intrusions. Hospital noise has negative effects, including sleep loss, heightened stress levels, elevated heart rate, and increased blood pressure. The constant beeping through hallway loudspeakers, paging systems, bells, alarms and staff voices bounce around the hard environmental surfaces creating a non-conducive healing atmosphere. Relaxing music, subliminal programming and guided imagery CD's can help create a more peaceful environment.

Physical Techniques

Stretching, yoga, and tai chi are examples of physical techniques used in complementary and alternative medicine. Tai chi, which originated in China as a martial art, is sometimes referred to as "moving meditation," as practitioners move their bodies slowly, gently, and with awareness, while breathing deeply. Tai chi incorporates the Chinese concepts of yin and yang, the concept of two opposing yet complementary forces described in traditional Chinese medicine. Yin represents cold, slow, or passive aspects of the person, while yang represents hot, excited, or active aspects. A major theory is that health is achieved through balancing yin and yang, and that disease is caused by an imbalance leading to a blockage in the flow of qi (pronounced, *chee*), Practicing tai chi supports a healthy balance of yin and yang, thereby aiding the flow of qi.

Research shows tai chi's potential for preventing falls, improving cardiovascular fitness, and improving overall well-being. Studies also looked at tai chi's possible benefits for a variety of other conditions, including hypertension and osteoarthritis and showed that tai chi reduced participants' blood pressure in twenty-two of twenty-six studies.

Hari Khalsa, MSN, FNP—a health care advocate and family nurse practitioner who runs Healthcare Whisperer in Waltham, Massachusetts—shared with me a simple way to make health care decisions with greater clarity. Hari says,

> When faced with the many unknowns of a health crisis or during times of stress, simple techniques from the ancient Kundalini Yoga tradition work to calm the body and settle the mind. These easy practices exist for all of us to use and help both the patient and the patient caregiver. The techniques are self-administered and their effects often surprisingly immediate and impactful. The "mind/body" connection is real.

> If you take a moment to think about the lungs and how they carry restorative oxygen through the blood to every body system and body tissue, then it is not a far leap to know that you can sooth, comfort your nerves and mind by simply working with

your own breath. When your mind and body are relaxed – greater clarity and better decision-making follow. (Khalsa, pers. comm.)

To experience greater peace and clarity, Hari suggests this breathing exercise:

For 3 minutes, sit in a chair, with your feet flat, spine straight and your eyes closed. Rest your hands, with palms up atop one another in your lap. Keep your chin slightly down and feel your body firmly supported but comfortably relaxed. Next, begin breathing in this simple 4 to 1 ratio. Inhale one complete breath in four equal strokes. Each stroke is a quick sniff through your nose. Gently hold this breath a few seconds in your chest, and then slowly exhale. This is one round. Repeat this pattern of breathing for the entire 3 minutes.

As you practice, observe the quality of your thoughts. Sometimes you may find your mind fully engaged in the patterned breathing. At other times, you may find your mind busily making plans or "in discussion." When this happens, kindly bring your focus back to the present experience of your breath in your body. To finish, inhale deeply. Fill your entire ribcage with breath. Then slowly exhale, smile, notice how you feel, and move on to enjoy your day.

Progressive Muscle Relaxation

Progressive muscle relaxation involves sequential tensing and relaxation of muscle groups—one at a time, progressing throughout the entire body. To practice progressive muscle relaxation, tense a group of muscles so they are as tightly contracted as possible. Hold them in a state of extreme tension for a few seconds. Then relax the muscles normally. Next, consciously relax the muscles even further so that you are as relaxed as possible. By tensing your muscles first, you will find that you are able to relax your muscles more than if you tried to relax your muscles directly. Start by relaxing the muscles in your legs and feet, working up through each muscle group to your neck, shoulders, and scalp.

Biofeedback

Biofeedback is another CAM technique in which you use your thoughts to control how your body functions, such as lowering your heart rate. With biofeedback, you are connected to electrical sensors that monitor your muscle tension, brain waves, or skin temperature. The information is sent back to you (feedback) to help to make subtle changes in your body (bio). By relaxing certain muscles, you learn how make physical changes in your body, including reducing pain.

Biofeedback has positive results on chemotherapy side effects, heart problems, asthma, high blood pressure, pain, and many other health related issues. Biofeedback may reduce or eliminate the need for medications, may be an option when medications haven't worked well, or may treat conditions during pregnancy when medications might be dangerous.

Acupuncture

Acupuncture, one of the oldest healing practices in the world, is a family of procedures involving the stimulation of specific points on the body using a variety of techniques, including penetrating the skin with needles that are then manipulated by hand or by electrical stimulation. Acupuncture is effective in treating a variety of medical conditions—respiratory disorders, disorders of the eye, osteoarthritis, nerve injury, heart related diseases, and it strengthens the immune system to help fight infections. Postsurgical nausea can also be reduced through acupuncture.

With certain health conditions, acupuncture can be effective enough to reduce or eliminate the need to take drugs to control pain. Acupuncture is available on a limited basis in a majority of teaching hospitals or outpatient clinics. If you are interested in receiving acupuncture during your hospital stay, ask your doctor to guide you.

Manipulative and Body-Based Practices

Manipulative and body-based practices focus primarily on the structures and systems of the body, including the bones and joints, soft tissues, and circulatory and lymphatic systems. Two commonly used therapies fall in this category:

1. *Spinal manipulation*—Chiropractors, physical therapists, osteo-paths, and some conventional medical doctors perform spinal manipulation. Practitioners use their hands or a device to apply a controlled force to a joint of the spine, moving it beyond its passive range of motion. The amount of force applied depends on the form of manipulation used. Spinal manipulation is among the treatment options used by people with low back pain—a very common condition that can be difficult to treat.

2. *Massage therapy*—the term *massage therapy* encompasses many different techniques. In general, therapists press, rub, and otherwise manipulate the muscles and other soft tissues of the body. People use massage for a variety of health-related purposes, including relieving pain, rehabilitating sports injuries, reducing stress, increasing relaxation, addressing anxiety and depression, and aiding general well-being.

CAM also encompasses movement therapies—a broad range of Eastern and Western movement-based approaches used to promote physical, mental, emotional, and spiritual well-being. Examples include Feldenkrais method, Alexander technique, Pilates, Rolfing, and Trager psychophysical integration. Reiki, magnet and light therapy, and qi gong are CAM practices that involve manipulation of energy fields.

Natural Products

This area of CAM includes use of a variety of herbal medicines (botanicals), vitamins, minerals, and other "natural products." Many are sold over the counter as dietary supplements. Natural products also include probiotics—live microorganisms (usually bacteria) that are similar to microorganisms normally found in the human digestive tract and may have beneficial effects. Probiotics are available in yogurts or as dietary supplements. Interest in natural products including omega 3 fish oils and echinacea have grown considerably in the past few decades.

Faith, Prayer, and Spirituality

Spirituality is an awareness of something greater than the individual self. It is often expressed through religion or prayer, although many other paths of spiritual quest and expression exist.

Many studies find that people with deep religious beliefs often enjoy positive outcomes after surgery. A new study presented at the American Psychological Association's 117th Annual Convention in Toronto found that people who have a deep reverence for life also enjoy that same benefit. The study looked at the effect of a range of faith factors, including traditional religious beliefs and practices and newer forms of spiritual seeking.

Researchers visited with one hundred and seventy-seven patients faced with coronary artery bypass graft surgery. They conducted interviews with the patients two weeks before their surgery dates to learn about their religious and secular spiritual beliefs and followed up with the patients after their surgeries. People who were spiritual in a secular way faced fewer postsurgery complications and didn't have to stay in the hospital as long as the patients who were not spiritual or religious. Reverence for life was the strongest of spirituality that helped patients.

Researchers found that frequency of prayer was also associated with fewer complications during recovery, whereas attendance at church was not. Almost every hospital includes spirituality and prayer as important components of healing. Hospitals also have chapels and arrangements with clergy and voluntary organizations to provide for patients' spiritual needs.

Prayer and beliefs, while not replacements for conventional medical care, are well worth pursuing, especially during a difficult medical time. Every evening before leaving the hospital, Bob, Kate, or Chris, and I stopped at the fountain in the atrium of the hospital. We searched our pockets for pennies, touched them together and softly chanted, "Gran, Gran, magical Gran, if she can't do it, nobody can." Then with belief and positive energy, we tossed the pennies into the water. Corny? Maybe— however it was our way of uniting the family in a solitary belief that Mom would survive.

On the critical morning when her external heart pump (RVAD) was scheduled for removal, the girls and I arrived to offer support. It was 5:00 AM, and her room was dark. Each girl took one of Mom's hands and one of my hands. No one spoke. Through this powerful ring, we circulated our strength and energy. Through our hands rushed common blood. It was a moving and powerful experience. Mom was sedated, yet in our hearts, we knew she was aware of our presence and our belief in her survival. The power of conviction, touch, and positive thoughts cannot be measured and should not be discounted.

Whole Medical Systems

Whole medical systems may be considered CAM. Examples of ancient whole medical systems include ayurvedic medicine and traditional Chinese medicine. Modern systems have developed in the past few centuries. Homeopathy, a whole medical system that originated in Europe, stimulates the body's ability to heal itself by giving very small doses of highly diluted substances that in larger doses would produce illness or symptoms. Naturopathy aims to support the body's ability to heal itself using dietary and lifestyle changes with herbs, massage, and joint **manipulation.**

Using CAM

As with any traditional medical treatment, if you decide to use CAM, take precautions to minimize risks.

Select CAM practitioners with care. Find out about the practitioner's training and experience. Be aware that dietary supplements may interact with medications or other supplements, may have side effects of their own, or may contain potentially harmful ingredients not listed on the label. Keep in mind that most supplements have not been tested in pregnant women, nursing mothers, or children.

When completing patient history forms, be sure to include all therapies and treatments you use. Tell your health care providers about any complementary and alternative practices you use. Give them a full picture of what you do to manage your health. This will help to ensure coordinated and safe care.

Do not use CAM as a replacement for conventional care, and do not postpone seeing a doctor about a medical problem. If you are considering a new CAM therapy, ask your health care providers about its safety, effectiveness, and possible interactions with medications, both prescription and nonprescription. If you have a medical condition or have not exercised in a while, consult with your health care provider before starting any CAM. Keep in mind that learning CAM techniques from a video or book does not ensure that you are doing the movements or learning the process correctly and safely.

Many CAM techniques can help shorten or even prevent a hospital stay if they are practiced regularly as part of a healthy and mindful lifestyle. In the hospital setting they are shown to do the following:

- decrease anxiety, pain and the use of medication for post-surgical pain
- reduce side effects of medical procedures and shorten recovery time and hospital stays
- allow for fewer complications and faster recovery
- strengthen the immune system
- help resist infections and improve healing
- increase sense of control and well-being
- improve decision making ability and enhance sleep
- reduce hospital expenses

Deep breathing exercises, meditation, and yoga rank among the top ten CAM practices. Progressive relaxation and guided imagery are also among the top CAM therapies for adults, while deep breathing and yoga ranked high among children. Begin today to incorporate the techniques and practices discussed in this chapter. Then, if a medical situation arises, you will be better equipped to survive the hospital stay as well as survive the illness.

CAM Resources

For more information on CAM, see the following websites:

- National Center for Complementary and Alternative Medicine at the National Institutes of Health (nccam.nih.gov)
- MedlinePlus—Complementary and Alternative Medicine (www.nlm.nih.gov/medlineplus/alternativemedicine.html)
- MedlinePlus—Herbs and Supplements (www.nlm.nih.gov/medlineplus/druginfo/herb_All.html)
- National Institutes of Health—Office of Dietary Supplements (www.ods.od.nih.gov)
- National Cancer Institute—Office of Cancer Complementary and Alternative Medicine (www.cancer.gov/cam)
- National Institute on Aging—Age Page on Dietary Supplements (www.nia.nih.gov/HealthInformation/ Publications/supplements.htm)

Final Thoughts

NOW is the time to face the truth and speak up about hospital safety. Trusting that a hospital is a safe harbor is a dangerous assumption. My mom suffered a severe myocardial infarction while in the recovery room after shoulder surgery. Her ECG reports showed a heart attack in progress many hours before emergency intervention.

Throughout the following months, the staff attempted to placate me by saying, "At least she was in the hospital when this happened." I disagree. A 911 call from home and an ambulance ride directly to the emergency room could have saved precious hours and heart muscle. Yet the hospital endeavored to reinforce the paradigm that she was in the best place possible to have a heart attack. Instead of owning up to their mistake, the hospital staff hoped to keep it from me. Because I had prior knowledge of the ECG results, their comments did little to soothe me. Honesty and an apology would have been appropriate.

Because of a hospital's blame-and-shame climate, no one admitted an error occurred, much less explained how it came to happen. I cannot help but wonder if the hospital used the adverse event to examine the reasons that caused it? Did they identify and change faulty protocols and procedures? Instead of hiding the mistake, could they have used it as an opportunity to reduce the chance of a reoccurrence? Except for bringing in additional revenue, did their error result in any good?

Mom's final hospital bills totaled more than $2 million. The hospital, doctors, surgeons, and specialists made massive amounts of money on the mistake the hospital caused. Where is the equity in that? I cannot think of another business model or situation where the damaged person pays the one who caused the damage. If someone crashes into your car and destroys your vehicle, do you pay them to fix it? And if you were forced to—could they possibly restore it back to its original condition? Sadly, the injured patient and family have no remedy except for a legal tug-of-war in an attempt to extract the truth. Lawsuits are lengthy, expensive, and unjust nonsolutions that ultimately do little to fix things for either party.

Throughout my research for this book, I interviewed patients, families, doctors, nurses, patient advocates, and anyone else who wanted to talk. Everyone had a story. My conversations ended with a universal consensus in favor of a patient-safety movement. Why? Because the system is defective. Drug companies create and perpetuate diseases. Hospitals function as corporations, and we accept their "kill them and bill them" business strategy. People treat doctors as demigods. Health care employees work beyond safe limits. Masking symptoms is the substitute for cures. Governing entities, drug companies, and politicians are in bed together, and the laws skew retribution. And each year, thousands of innocent patients continue to pay the price with their lives.

If we continue to approach a hospital stay as we have in the past, with complete surrender and faith, we cannot expect different or better outcomes. Nothing changes if nothing changes. To modify this paradigm, we must first understand it and then take action.

There is no doubt that every hospital patient needs an advocate. I hope this book jolts you out of complacency, gives you the information to understand the problems, and inspires you to become a force of change by creating your own hospital experience. Join me in our grassroots campaign to build an informed advocacy support group inside every club, organization, business, and community. Together—each of us can make a difference. You are well on your way to becoming a speak up and stay alive advocate for yourself or a loved one.

Do you have an Infection Protection Survival Bag?

One week before this book went to print, I had the opportunity to spend two days in the hospital with my mom. One of the sternal wound wires from her heart surgery poked through her skin and a staph infection developed. She was admitted, not only to remove the offending wire, but also to get the infection under control. As her advocate, I packed a bag filled with items to disinfect the room—and other comforting necessities.

Armed with my knowledge shared in this book, I entered her hospital room like a hazmat responder. I donned a pair of gloves, grabbed my container of disinfectant wipes and began my cleaning frenzy. Because C diff survives most disinfectants, I also sprayed every surface with a bleach and water solution, paying extra attention to the bathroom. I checked the mattress for signs of bed bugs, (yes, they live in hospitals too). I disinfected the call button and the TV remote and wrapped the remote with a plastic protector found in the Patient Pod. I covered the dingy hospital pillow with a clean and pretty, handmade pillowcase from home. (After Mom's initial heart surgery, she could not go back to work, so she gives back by making beautiful pillowcases. We send them to our troops overseas and use them for other charitable fundraisers.) I even remembered the radiant health CD she likes so much. Once the room was prepared, we were ready to concentrate on getting well and getting out.

My bag of supplies made me think of how other patients approach their room upon hospital admission. Most people get to the room, take off their clothes, shoes and socks, put on a flimsy gown and hop into bed with bare feet that touched the dirty floor. Next they put eyeglasses, cell phones, and other personal items on a germ laden bedside table, reach for the bacteria rich TV remote or call button, adjust the bed with the push buttons recently used by the previous sick person, and rest their head on an unfamiliar pillow. Thoroughly covered with infectious pathogens, they begin their hospital journey at a disadvantage. These thoughts inspired me to devise the Infection Protection Survival Bag. This bag contains most of the items you need to disinfect your room and help keep you safe and comfortable while in the hospital. Some of the goodies in the bag include:

- A copy of the book, Speak Up and Stay Alive
- The Patient Safety Logs, a Clean Your Hands sign, a medical terminology guide and more
- The Patient Pod
- A Radiant Health or Healing CD
- A "Positively Pocket Pillowcase" with a positive affirmation card. (Mom's handmade pillowcase with a small pocket that holds a card engraved with positive health suggestions. Read the positive affirmations just before falling asleep, and then tuck the card back into the pillowcase pocket. All through the night, your subconscious mind works to make those thoughts a reality.)
- A container of disinfectant wipes
- Two disposable gloves

The bag is large enough to add your personal items. Everyone should have a prepared hospital bag. When a health crisis strikes, you may not have the luxury of time or clear thinking. Having a pre-packed infection protection bag makes it easy to stay safe should you or a loved one encounter a hospital stay.

The Infection Protection Survival Bag—filled with vital necessities for your safety and well-being is available: www.speakupandstayalive.com

Speak Up and Stay Alive
Patricia J. Rullo
46 Chagrin Plaza #103
Chagrin Falls, Ohio
440-725-5462
www.speakupandstayalive.com
pat@speakupandstayalive.com

For information about the pocket pillowcases: www.pillowcase4u.com
To view our troops and veterans efforts: www.sewportourtroops.com
To use our pillowcases as a fundraiser for your group:
www.acaseforacause.com

Helping Hands

THE following health care navigators and patient advocates are included for your convenience. Each of the dedicated women listed in this Helping Hands section are educated, experienced and committed to help you survive a hospital stay. Please reach out to them when you need help.

When You Need Help

An advocate is an important tool that patients can use when they feel they have reached an impasse with the healthcare system. As a patient care coordinator, we can step up and provide support for you.

Are you feeling overwhelmed trying to manage your chronic illness? We can speak with your medical team if you are unclear about a diagnosis or new medication as well as organize transportation for appointments.

Do you need to choose an assisted living or nursing home for a loved one? We can assist you with the selection process. Once we know your needs, we will research and assess the potential facilities in your area and compile a comprehensive list of potential nursing homes that meet your requirements.

Are you overwhelmed by your health insurance? If you have questions on what you owe or you need to appeal a denial, help is near at hand. We can also help you find new insurance that fits your needs.

Is your primary care physician or specialist not paying attention to your concerns? We can help locate a new physician or specialist to better suit your needs. We can also help locate specialty treatment centers, should you require further medical care.

If your needs and concerns are not being met, we will help guide you to get what you need. We never lose sight of the fact that the patient is the most important person in the room.

Healthcare Whisperer
Hari Khalsa - Healthcare Advocate & Family Nurse Practitioner
Founder and Owner
785 Beaver Street, Waltham, MA 02452
Phone: 866-980-4325
www.healthcarewhisperer.com
heal@healthcarewhisperer.com
The Empowered Radio Show

Why Engage a Healthcare Navigation Specialist?

1. Because our healthcare system is broken putting you at risk physically, emotionally and financially. Our healthcare navigation specialists are trained to listen to and support you on every needed level; whatever your situation. We stand by you, and always keep a strong focus on total quality of your health, life and well-being.

2. Because you won't always get referred to the best physicians or hospital. Physicians often limit their referrals to their own networks. We find you the right and best doctors and treatment facilities, whoever and wherever they are.

3. Because being in the hospital exposes you to serious risks. We help you stay out of the hospital, or help you minimize your risks if you have to go there. Our healthcare navigation specialists provide active guidance on how to stay safe, avoid complications and errors while you're in any medical facility, and improve your chances for a fast release.

    It takes an insider to help you move through it. Engage one of our healthcare navigation specialists, who will spend time with you one-on-one to understand you and your needs, and assist you in reaching a plan of action consistent with your goals, beliefs and comfort level.

    Livingwell Care Navigation works with private clients worldwide, providing personal guidance and support from prevention and lifestyle management of chronic disorders to elder care, medical crisis intervention and ultimately, easeful dying.

Livingwell Care Navigation Inc.
Barbara Abruzzo RN
Founder and Owner
Phone: 646-820-6556
www.livingwellcarenavigation.com
info@ livingwellcarenavigation.com

Reach Your Personal Health Outcomes

GOLDEN NAVIGATOR helps others face the challenges the health care environment creates. With a compassionate ear and the skills to find resources and answers, GOLDEN NAVIGATOR can:

- Accompany you or loved one to physician appointments, formulate questions and help follow-up on health recommendations.
- Help review medical bills, appeal unpaid claims and obtain pre-authorization for treatments.
- Coordinate health care procedures, treatments and plans.
- Develop a personal health record for emergencies and health-care appointments.
- Educate on alternative ways to achieve your personal health-care goals.
- Advocate on your behalf with physicians and hospital staff.
- Review medical records for accuracy and assist with obtaining second opinions.
- Explore health treatment options and guide your decision-making.
- Assist with discharge planning, assessment of needs and medication reconciliation.
- Educate on safety issues, living arrangements, and issues in regards to memory loss in the geriatric clients.
- Help with the transition from the hospital to a rehabilitation facility, skilled nursing facility or home.
- Develop personal health management tools for your medications and specific health conditions.

Karen Morrisey has over thirty years in the healthcare arena. She ended her full time vocation to tend to the complex medical needs of her parents, husband and other loved ones. As a patient advocate, Karen incorporates the NAHAC Code of Ethics into her daily practice and offers her clients a customized approach to help reach their personal health outcomes.

GOLDEN NAVIGATOR
The Gold Standard in Patient Advocacy
Karen Morrisey
HealthCare Consultant
Phone: 480-421-9265 (o)
Phone: 602-363-0240 (c)
Fax: 480-699-5790
GoldenNavigator@cox.net

Increase Your Quality Time

Caring for a sick loved one is very personal. Every situation is different. The little things that matter make a very big difference. Yet there are so many details, that families have little quality time with their loved ones. To insure you receive the ultimate level of care when you need it most and to offer respite for caretakers, we will:

- Asses your situation, gather personal and medical information and discuss your needs and immediate problems to provide the right solutions.
- Research and review your healthcare records or help acquire them from the relevant hospital or physician.
- Discuss with you and your healthcare providers about recommended treatments and coordinate efforts among all medical service providers.
- Investigate all types of insurance, facilitate changes or reinstate your insurance coverage as well as file and follow up on forms necessary to guarantee continuous coverage.
- Assist with medication management such as proper dosing and coordinating refills with physicians and area pharmacies.
- Help with environmental changes such as hospital check in, room set-up, arranging for comforts and necessities, establishing relationships with key staff to brief them on your needs, routines, medical care and family expectations.
- Support hospice and end of life care to keep you or your loved one dignified and comfortable during this sensitive time.

Carol provides compassionate and professional advocacy services on behalf of patients and their families. She liaises with insurance companies, physicians, pharmacies, extended care facilities and clinicians to provide the highest level of care and consistency between providers. As part of her comprehensive care package, Carol spends time with patients, supplying comfort, peace of mind and emotional support.

C. Cleary Cusick, Inc.
Carol Cusick, Founder
154 Martling Avenue
Tarrytown, New York 10591
Phone: 914-588-7940
www.cclearycusick.com
carol@cclearycusick.com

Helping Seniors Navigate Life's Next Step

Change is stressful for everyone, but for older adults, it can be particularly difficult. How to navigate the next step can seem overwhelming. If you or someone you care for is experiencing an abrupt health-related change that requires immediate accommodation, is planning ahead to live independently, is coping with a chronic condition or if you are just concerned about their well-being, you may need an experienced nurse advocate to help manage their care and provide highly personalized help to:

- Coordinate and manage care throughout an illness
- Advocate and supervise quality of care
- Act as a liaison between family and medical staff
- Promote independence at home by offering recommendations to address individual needs and safety concerns
- Adapt home to accommodate needs
- Provide referrals for community services, in-home healthcare services and procurement of healthcare equipment, supplies and resources as needed.
- Select the right assisted living or nursing home community if needed
- Attend family meetings to review care plan and advocate for your family member's needs
- Address concerns about a loved one's well-being and care
- Make sure your loved one receives the quality care he or she needs, whether living independently, at home or in an assisted living or nursing home community.

Tracey's 20 years of experience in nursing and volunteer work as a Certified Long Term Care Ombudsman for the State of Massachusetts have reinforced her determination to improve the lives of seniors by providing expertise and support.

Transition with Care - Senior Advocates
Tracey Driscoll, RN, MHA
P.O. Box 503
Concord, MA 01742
Phone: 1-800-933-1592
www.transitionwithcare.com
tdriscoll@transitionwithcare.com

How to Control Medical Costs

- How do you determine reasonable medical fees?
- Do you know how to negotiate with your insurance carrier for out of network services and deductibles?
- Are you overpaying your claims?
- How can you detect potential fraud?

Insurance fraud costs the insurance industry nearly $100 billion dollars per year. Anti-fraud programs can safeguard you against unnecessary and inappropriate medical and chiropractic care and expense. This service applies for all lines of business: Workers' Compensation, Auto, Group Health and Liability. By using a three-step process, we identify, establish and report unnecessary and inappropriate services. We review and summarize the medical or chiropractic records and then compare the treatment to standard medical protocols. Medical or Chiropractic doctors provide their independent professional opinion about the treatment rendered. Next, a financial analysis includes both bill review and clinical review reductions. This independent review provides clients with an easy to read report that clearly identifies unnecessary and inappropriate services that can be forwarded to their Special Investigations Unit or to the State for further investigation.

Professional bill review, medical and chiropractic reviews, and investigations to identify over-treatment and over-billing as well as fraud and abuse are ways to positively impact your bottom line.

Medical Cost Control Inc. is an independently owned, disabled veteran founded enterprise with a nationwide reputation for excellence in medical and chiropractic cost containment services. MCCI provides bill review and fee negotiations services across all 50 states with customized processes to meet clients' individual needs.

Medical Cost Control Inc.
Tricia Ruminski
930 Gleneagles Rd.
Beaumont, CA 92223
Phone: 909-385-4600 ext 722
Fax: 951-769-3630
www.medicalcostcontrol.com
tricia.ruminski@medicalcostcontrol.com

Patient Advocacy, Wellness, and Pain Management

- Are you confused about the information your doctor has provided?
- Do you suffer from chronic stress or pain?
- Do you feel rushed during doctor appointments?
- Do you need someone on your side to fight for you and your rights?

A patient advocate can provide you and your family the proper guidance, support, and education to resolve these care challenges and more. As a patient advocate, I can:

- Help prevent medical mistakes, including hospital-acquired infections
- Monitor you bedside while you are hospitalized
- Help manage chronic pain
- Assist with mental preparation for surgery, treatments, procedures, chemotherapy, and radiation
- Assist with veteran's benefits
- Lower costs by reducing unnecessary physician visits

Services focused on seniors include:

- Management of medications and prevention of overmedication
- Prevention of unnecessary treatment
- Decreasing hospital readmissions

Linda uses her 30 years experience as a patient-focused medical professional and her Masters Degree in Gerontology, to assist individuals and families with their health care challenges. From developing a treatment plan, to tackling health insurance issues, coaching wellness practices and guiding patients to overcome chronic pain issues, Linda is available to help you weather whatever health challenges you encounter.

Patient Advocate Bay Area, Inc
Linda Garvin, RN, MSN
Nurse Patient Advocate
Phone: 510-520-0186
Fax: 510-523-3774
www.patientadvocatebayarea.com
www.lindagarvin.com
linda@healthadvocatebayarea.com

A Simple, Sensible Health Solution

The all-new Patient Pod is a "Portable Wellness Center" created to answer these questions:

- How are bedridden patients supposed to clean their hands?
- Is there a safe, clean, and accessible place for a patient's cell phone, eyeglasses, or hearing aids, so they don't get damaged, lost, or moved out of reach?
- Is there a way for patients and caregivers to communicate using a low-tech messaging system?
- How can patients become empowered, proactive, safer, and satisfied?

The Patient Pod is that solution. It's a personal storage system coupled to a unique, swiveling attachment clamp. It attaches to the bed rail and keeps personal items within reach, while reducing germ transfer at the bedside. It lowers the risk of hospital-acquired infections and patient falls, reduces caregiver steps, and helps manage discharge materials.

The Patient Pod comes pre-packaged with

- Hand sanitizer
- Sanitizing wipes
- A custom cover (plus a spare) for the germiest item in the room - the TV remote control
- A notepad and pen
- Six essential tips on how to partner with caregivers and guard against infection.

The "face" of the Patient Pod displays your personal photo and preferred name and you can post a message in the integrated clip (alerting caregivers to an allergy or a hearing problem, for instance). These features help caregivers communicate and engage with you. When you leave the hospital or nursing home, the Pod travels with you on your walker, wheelchair, chair rail, seat back, or baby stroller.

Some say having a Patient Pod is "like bringing a friend to the hospital with you; familiar and comforting…in a place where nothing you touch is yours."

Pear Health LLC - Makers of The Patient Pod
Pat Mastors
Founder and CEO
5700 Post Rd., Suite 300
East Greenwich, RI 02818
Phone: 1-855-55 PATIENT (1-855-557-2843)
www.thepatientpod.com
pmastors@thepatientpod.com

References

American Academy of Pediatrics. 1999. *The relationship between perceived parental expectations and pediatrician antimicrobial prescribing behavior.*

American Hospital Association. 2003. *The Patient Care Partnership— Understanding Expectations, Rights and Responsibilities.* www.aha.org/advocacy-issues/communicatingpts/pt-care-partnership. shtml.

B.D. Eckstein et al. MBC Infectious Diseases 2007, 7 :61.

American Society for Microbiology. 2006. *Ventilator-Associated Pneumonia: Diagnosis, Treatment, and Prevention.* www.ncbi.nlm.nih.gov/pmc/articles/PMC1592694/

Annals of Family Medicine, Inc. 2007. *Creating Demand for Prescription Drugs: A Content Analysis of Television Direct-to-Consumer Advertising.* www.annfammed.org/content/5/1/6.full

Annals of Internal Medicine. 2003. *The Incidence and Severity of Adverse Events Affecting Patients after Discharge from the Hospital.* www.annals.org/content/138/3/161.full.pdf+html

Annals of Internal Medicine. 2011. "July Effect": Impact of the Academic Year-End Changeover on Patient Outcomes. A Systematic Review. www.annals.org/search?fulltext=2011+july+effect&submit=yes

Centers for Disease Control and Prevention. 2009. *Guideline for Prevention of Catheter-Associated Urinary Tract Infections.*
www.cdc.gov/hicpac/pdf/CAUTI/CAUTIguideline2009final.pdf

Centers for Disease Control and Prevention. 2003. *Guidelines for Preventing Health-care Associated Pneumonia.*
www.cdc.gov/hicpac/pdf/guidelines/HApneu2003guidelines.pdf

Centers for Disease Control and Prevention. 2011. *Hand Hygiene Brochure.*
www.cdc.gov/handhygiene/PDF/CDC_HandHygiene_Brochure.pdf

Centers for Disease Control and Prevention. 2011. *Infection Prevention during Blood Glucose Monitoring and Insulin Administration.*
www.cdc.gov/injectionsafety/blood-glucose-monitoring.html

Centers for Disease Control and Prevention. 2011. *Information for Patients – Injection Safety.*
www.cdc.gov/injectionsafety/patients.html

Committee to Reduce Infection Deaths. 2011. *Hospital infection is the next asbestos.*
www.hospitalinfection.org/nextasbestos.shtml

Department of Health and Human Services. 2010. *Adverse Events in Hospitals: National Incidence Among Medicare Beneficiaries.*
OEI-06-09-00090
http://oig.hhs.gov/oei/reports/oei-06-09-00090.pdf

Endometriosis.org. 2011.
http://endometriosis.org/news/support-awareness/
endometriosis-awareness-week-creates-noise-light-and-hope/

Hysterectomy Educational Resources and Services. 2011. *HERS Foundation's Adverse Effects Data Bank.*

www.hersfoundation.com/take_action.htm

Infection Control Today. 2011
www.infectioncontroltoday.com/Webinars.aspx

Institute for Safe Medication Practices. 2009. *ISMP Medication Safety Alert Acute Care.* (ISSN 1550-6312) 2009
www.whackamolethebook.com/wp-content/uploads/2011/09/ismp09newsletter.pdf

Institute of Medicine. 2006. *Preventing Medication Errors.*
http://iom.edu/~/media/Files/Report%20Files/2006/Preventing-Medication-Errors-Quality-Chasm-Series/medicationerrorsnew.ashx

Institute of Medicine. 1999. *To Err is Human, Building a Safer Health System.*
www.iom.edu/~/media/Files/Report%20Files/1999/To-Err-is-Human/To%20Err%20is%20Human%201999%20%20report%20brief.pdf

Journal of Hospital Infection. 2004. *National Clostridium difficile Standards Group: Report to the Department of Health.*
(Vol. 56Supplement 1, Pages 1-38, DOI: 10.1016/j.jhin.2003.10.016)
www.journalofhospitalinfection.com/article/S0195-6701(03)00433-X/fulltext

National Alliance for Caregiving. 2010. *Caregivers of Veterans – Serving on the Homefront.*
www.caregiving.org/archives/1686
www.caregiving.org/data/2010_Caregivers_of_Veterans_FULLREPORT_WEB_FINAL.pdf

National Center for Health. 2011. *Use of advance directives in long-term care populations.*
www.cdc.gov/nchs/data/databriefs/db54.htm

National Center for Missing & Exploited Children. 2009. *Guidelines on Prevention of and Response to Infant Abductions.*
www.missingkids.com/en_US/publications/NC05.pdf

National Heart, Lung, and Blood Institute. 2005. *Facts about Menopausal Hormone Therapy.*
www.nhlbi.nih.gov/health/women/pht_facts.pdf

National Heart, Lung and Blood Institute. 2007. *The Healthy Heart Handbook for Women.*
www.nhlbi.nih.gov/health/public/heart/other/hhw/hdbk_wmn.pdf

National Patient Safety Foundation. 2003. *The Role of the Patient Advocate—A Consumer Fact Sheet.*
www.npsf.org/pdf/paf/PatientAdvocate.pdf

National Quality Forum. 2011. *Safe Practices for Better Healthcare.*
www.qualityforum.org/News_And_Resources/Press_Kits/Safe_
Practices_for_Better_Healthcare.aspx

New England Journal of Medicine. 2011. *Nurse Staffing and Inpatient Hospital Mortality.*
www.truthaboutnursing.org/news/2011/mar/orig/16_twincities.html

New England Journal of Medicine. 2009. *Rehospitalizations among patients in the Medicare fee-for-service program.*
www.nejm.org/doi/full/10.1056/NEJMsa0803563

New England Journal of Medicine. 2011. *Restrictions on the Use of Prescribing Data for Drug Promotion.*
www.nejm.org/doi/pdf/10.1056/NEJMhle1107678

The American Cancer Society. 2011. *What are the key statistics about ovarian cancer?*
www.cancer.org/Cancer/OvarianCancer/DetailedGuide/
ovarian-cancer-key-statistics

The American Journal of Geriatric Psychiatry. 2010. *Interactions Cause Seniors to Drop Anti-depressants.*
www.reuters.com/article/2010/12/17/
us-interactions-antidepressants-idUSTRE6BG63T20101217

The Joint Commission. 2011. *FAQs on radiation overdose.*
www.jointcommission.org/sentinel_event.aspx

The Joint Commission. 2010. *Joint Commission Center for Transforming Healthcare*
Press Conference for Hand-off Communications.
www.centerfortransforminghealthcare.org/news/press/handoff.aspx

The Joint Commission. 2010. *Sentinel Event 45. Alert Preventing violence in the health care setting.*
www.jointcommission.org/assets/1/18/SEA_45.PDF www.
jointcommission.org/sentinel_event_alert_issue_45_preventing_
violence_in_the_health_care_setting_/

The Joint Commission. 2010. *Sentinel Event Alert 46. Focus on medical/surgical units and the emergency department.*
www.jointcommission.org/sentinel_event_alert_issue_46_a_follow-up_
report_on_preventing_suicide_focus_on_medicalsurgical_units_and_
the_emergency_department/

The Joint Commission. 2011. *Sentinel Event Data - Event Type by Year; Sentinel Event Data - Root Causes by Event Type.*
www.jointcommission.org/sentinel_event.aspx

The Joint Commission. 2011. *Speak Up: Prevent Errors in Your Child's Care.*
www.jointcommission.org/
Speak_Up_Prevent_Errors_in_Your_Childs_Care/

The Joint Commission. 2007. *What Did the Doctor Say? Improving Health Literacy to Protect Patient Safety*
www.jointcommission.org/What_Did_the_Doctor_Say/

The Journal of the American Medical Association. 2001. *Medication Errors in Children.*
http://jama.ama-assn.org/content/285/16/2114

Pro-Stat®. 2011. *Pro-Stat® in the treatment of pressure ulcers.*
www.pro-stat.info/pro-stat_indication_press.asp

Resources

How to evaluate medical websites

USE your favorite search engine and type in a disease or medical condition. Do you find hundreds of choices? How do you know which sites offer reliable information? To lessen the amount of sites that may not contain applicable information, narrow your search. If you want advice on a heart condition, be specific. If you type in "heart disease," you find links to general information about a broad range of heart issues. Refine your search and enter "heart failure" or "heart valve disease," and you obtain targeted links with specific information.

Now that your selection is relevant, how do you determine reliability? The web address can provide a clue. A professional organization uses ".org" in their address. A ".gov" is for government agencies. An address ending in ".edu" indicates an educational institution and ".com" is generally used for commercial sites. Look to see who funds the site, the purpose of the site and the source. Many websites have an "About" page that shares information about the founders and their mission. Many commercial sites offer valuable and credible information while others represent companies selling products. While a site that promotes products may have honest information, continue searching other sites to verify that information. Medical websites may be geared to health professionals, to consumers, or to both. Many professional health care sites are loaded with medical lingo yet are also rich in content. Use these sites in conjunction with government, educational and commercial sites. To make sure the data is current, check the bottom of the page for a revision date.

Opinions, consumer blogs, threads and forums are interesting and may offer suggestions and solutions not found in traditional sources. For instance, if you find multiple consumer forums complaining about a drug side effect, use that piece of information as a new search word or phrase. This can lead to additional verifiable sources. Using the Internet is similar to detective work. Gather clues, check multiple resources, and work with your health care providers to create a solution.

The following are websites in the order they appear in the book. The contact details are accurate as of the book's publication date. However, information may change and the websites may no longer be available or have different addresses. Do not construe the use of these or any websites as substitutes for qualified medical advice from trained and credentialed professionals.

Speak Up and Stay Alive
www.speakupandstayalive.com
A hospital survival guide published by Millennium Star Publishing
    to help save patients and their advocates from today's
    dangerous health care.

National Association of Health Advocacy Consultants (NAHAC)
www.nahac.com
Locate a health care advocate

AdvoConnection
www.advoconnection.com
Locate a health care advocate *in Health Care Assistance*

The American Medical Association
www.ama-assn.org
Research doctor's education, certification and performance history

The American Board of Medical Specialties
www.abms.org
Research doctor's education, certification and performance history

Patients Right to Know.org
www.patientsrighttoknow.org

Go to your state's physician licensing website to check for any
license revocation history

American College of Surgeons
www.facs.org
Find a doctor or a surgeon.

The Joint Commission
www.jcaho.org
Find out if your hospital is accredited. An independent, not-for-
profit organization, The Joint Commission accredits and
certifies more than 19,000 health care organizations and
programs in the United States.

Accreditation Organization for Ambulatory Healthcare
www.aaahc.org
Accredits almost 5,000 organizations in a wide variety of ambulatory health care settings, including ambulatory and surgery
centers, community health centers, medical and dental group
practices, medical home, and managed care organizations, as
well as Indian and student health centers, among others. They
are also the official accrediting organization for the US Air
Force and the US Coast Guard.

Hospital Compare
www.hospitalcompare.hhs.gov
Compare your hospital with others. This website from the
Department of Health and Human Services allows you to
search by city, state or other criteria and look up statistics
comparing more than 5,000 hospitals against one another and
to state and federal averages.

The National Quality Forum
www.qualityforum.org
Advances efforts to improve quality through performance measurement and public reporting

Institute for Safe Medication Practices

www.ismp.org/

The Institute for Safe Medication Practices (ISMP) is devoted to
    medication error prevention and safe medication use.

For a list of error prone medication abbreviations:

www.ismp.org/tools/errorproneabbreviations.pdf

For a list of high alert medications:

www.ismp.org/tools/highalertmedications.pdf

Infection Control Today

www.infectioncontroltoday.com

Infection Control Today magazine, website and e-newsletters
    deliver timely, relevant guidance that medical professionals
    need to protect their institutions, patients and fellow health
    care workers, and to eliminate health care-acquired infections.
    Interesting articles and webinars.

The Consumer Reports

www.consumerreports.org

Lists hospital ratings by state

Centers for Medicare and Medicaid Services

www.cms.gov

Lots of tools, resources, statistics and consumer information

    The American Foundation for Suicide Prevention

www.afsp.org

National Suicide Prevention Lifeline

www.suicidepreventionlifeline.org

The Veterans Crisis Line

www.veteranscrisisline.net

Connects Veterans in crisis and their families and friends with

qualified, caring Department of Veterans Affairs responders
through a confidential toll-free hotline and online chat

American Diabetes Association
www.diabetes.org

Ovarian Cancer National Alliance
www.ovariancancer.org

National Ovarian Cancer Coalition
www.ovarian.org

United States Department of Veteran Affairs
www.caregiver.va.gov
www.myhealth.va.gov

MedlinePlus—Complementary and Alternative Medicine
www.nlm.nih.gov/medlineplus/alternativemedicine.html

MedlinePlus—Herbs and Supplements
www.nlm.nih.gov/medlineplus/druginfo/herb_All.html

National Institutes of Health—Office of Dietary Supplements
(ODS)
http://ods.od.nih.gov
Supports research on dietary supplements, distributes the results
of research on dietary supplements and provides educational
material on dietary supplements, including fact sheets and other
reliable health information.

National Cancer Institute—Office of Cancer Complementary and
Alternative Medicine
www.cancer.gov/cam
Coordinates and enhances the activities of the National Cancer
Institute (NCI) in the arena of complementary and alternative
medicine (CAM).

National Institute on Aging (NIA)

www.nia.nih.gov

Provides leadership in aging research, training, health information dissemination and other programs relevant to aging and older people

National Institute on Aging—Age Page on Dietary Supplements www.nia.nih.gov/HealthInformation/ Publications/supplements. htm

About the Author

PAT is a nationally known speaker and coach in the insurance and banking industry and has served on the advisory boards of New York Life Insurance Company and Transamerica Life Insurance Company. She is recognized through Consulting Psychologists Press as a certified administrator and interpreter of the Myers-Briggs Type Indicator, an assessment instrument that provides in-depth insights into personality type and behavior. She is the author of many business magazine articles and the books - Worksite Marketing—A Promise to Deliver, Succeed with Style and When Daddy Plays Golf. Pat and her mom founded the charity Sewport Our Troops and the charitable fundraising company, A Case for a Cause. Pat also makes time for daily contemplation in her pink kayak at her summer home on the Chagrin River in Ohio and desert tai chi at her winter home in the Superstition Mountains of Arizona.

In conjunction with the book, *Speak Up and Stay Alive*, Pat educates groups, clubs, organizations, and businesses about the hazards of hospital stays, how to survive them and the importance of having a health care advocate.

You can join the Speak Up and Stay Alive patient safety and advocacy movement. Here's how:

1. Educate and empower your group, club or employees. Schedule the author as a guest speaker. Topics can be tailored to your crowd. The presentation is jam packed with serious information, delivered with a light touch of wit and humor.
2. Share your hospital story in an upcoming book, Speak Up and Stay Alive – Patients & Advocates Tell All.
3. Start a Speak Up and Stay Alive affiliate in your city, club, business, or organization. Allow your members or employees to

appreciate the need for a hospital advocate. Build a ready-to-take-action support group within your existing group. When a member of your organization goes to the hospital, your Speak Up and Stay Alive advocacy group will be prepared to help out. The author will work with your members and make the book, the safety logs, and the infection protection bags available to you.

Pat says, "This book is only a vehicle to share information. It cannot take action by itself. As the reader, you have the power to alter the path of hospital safety. I encourage you to integrate your new knowledge within your circle of influence. If each of us helps one other person survive a hospital stay, then this book is doing its job."

Patricia J. Rullo
www.speakupandstayalive.com
speak@speakupandstayalive.com
440-725-5462

Index